Advance Praise for
Fit Nurse: Your Total Plan for Getting Fit and Living Well

"*Fit Nurse: Your Total Plan for Getting Fit and Living Well* is an interactive book that encourages healthcare professionals to design and own their personal plan of care. Reading about similar experiences from others in my profession allowed me to be honest with my own lifestyle assessment. I applaud Gary Scholar. He is a true advocate for the health and wellness of nurses."

–Cathy Clark, RN
Night Shift Liaison
AtlantiCare Regional Medical Center
Pomona, New Jersey

"As caregivers, nurses are keenly aware of healthy versus unhealthy lifestyles, but often find it difficult to incorporate these strategies into their own hectic lives. *Fit Nurse: Your Total Plan for Getting Fit and Living Well* clearly identifies the challenges nurses face and offers the encouragement, inspiration, and support to incorporate these healthy choices into your lifestyle. This book takes the work out of doing what you know you need to do for yourself, but might not know how to get started. There's even a chapter dedicated to the specific needs of working the night shift. The interactive style of the book plugs you right into the content, so keep a notepad and pen handy (or write notes in your book) . . . and you are on your way! Do this for you. You deserve it!

–Eileen Gallen Bademan, RN, BSN
Staff Nurse
St. Mary Medical Center
Langhorne, Pennsylvania
Author of *A Daybook for Critical Care Nurses*

FIT
NURSE

Your Total Plan for
Getting Fit and Living Well

Gary Scholar, M.Ed.

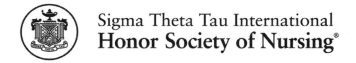

Sigma Theta Tau International
Honor Society of Nursing®

Sigma Theta Tau International

Copyright © 2010 by Sigma Theta Tau International

All rights reserved. This book is protected by copyright. No part of it may be reproduced, stored in a retrieval system, or transmitted in any form or by any means, electronic, mechanical, photocopying, recording, or otherwise, without written permission from the publisher.

Any trademarks, service marks, design rights, or similar rights that are mentioned, used, or cited in this book are the property of their respective owners. Their use here does not imply that you may use them for similar or any other purpose.

Sigma Theta Tau International
550 West North Street
Indianapolis, IN 46202

To order additional books, buy in bulk, or order for corporate use, contact Nursing Knowledge International at 888.NKI.4YOU (888.654.4968/US and Canada) or +1.317.634.8171 (outside US and Canada).

To request a review copy for course adoption, e-mail solutions@nursingknowledge.org or call 888.NKI.4YOU (888.654.4968/US and Canada) or +1.317.917.4983 (outside US and Canada).

To request author information, or for speaker or other media requests, contact Rachael McLaughlin of the Honor Society of Nursing, Sigma Theta Tau International at 888.634.7575 (US and Canada) or +1.317.634.8171 (outside US and Canada).

ISBN-13: 978-1-930538-94-8

Library of Congress Cataloging-in-Publication Data

Scholar, Gary, 1955-
  Fit nurse : your total plan for getting fit and living well / Gary Scholar.
    p. ; cm.
  Includes bibliographical references.
  ISBN 978-1-930538-94-8
  1. Nurses--Health and hygiene. 2. Physical fitness. I. Sigma Theta Tau International. II. Title.
  [DNLM: 1. Nurses. 2. Physical Fitness. QT 255 S368f 2010]
  RT67.S36 2010
  610.73--dc22
                          2009048674

First Printing, 2010

Publisher: Renee Wilmeth
Acquisitions Editor: Cynthia Saver, RN, MS
Editorial Coordinator: Paula Jeffers
Cover Designer: Rebecca Batchelor
Interior Design and Page Composition: Rebecca Batchelor

Principal Editor: Carla Hall
Copy Editor: Kevin Kent
Proofreader: Billy Fields
Indexer: Johnna VanHoose Dinse
Illustrator: Rebecca Batchelor

Dedication

This book is dedicated to my mom, Rita Scholar, who always wanted to be a nurse, but life circumstances led her down a different path. Still, she realized part of her dream by volunteering at a hospital for 15 years.

To my dad, Edward Scholar, and my mom who constantly encouraged me in my writing.

To nurse executive Karen Hendrickson of Southeast Missouri Hospital, who inspired me with her commitment of self-care for a healthier lifestyle.

To all nurses, who are inspirational, compassionate heroes.

Cover photo credits: (Back, from L-R: photo 1 and author photo by Kaiti Green of James Photo Studio, Chicago, Illinois; photo 2 from istockphoto.com; photo 3 by Jane Palmer, Sigma Theta Tau International, Indianapolis, Indiana. Front top by Kaiti Green of James Photo Studio, Chicago, Illinois; middle from istockphoto.com; bottom by Kaiti Green of James Photo Studio, Chicago, Illinois.)

Acknowledgements

This book would not have been possible without the support, encouragement, and inspiration from so many people. I want to express my special thanks to the following people:

Raina Childers, RD, director of Health Point Fitness

Roseann Kobialka, director of organizational development, AtlantiCare

Robyn Begley, DNP, RN, CNEA-BC, vice president of nursing/CNO, AtlantiCare

Cathy Clark, RN, night shift liaison, AtlantiCare Regional Medical Center

All the amazing nurses at AtlantiCare

All the nurses who so willingly shared their stories for this book

Karen Hendrickson, nurse executive at Southeast Missouri Hospital, Cape Girardeau, Missouri

Caroline Jung

Karen Redmond

Mona Wu

Rhonda Fentry

Kaiti Green, photographer, James Photo Studio

Grace Walker (the meditating RN in scrubs on the back cover) and Kelly Sego of Clarian Health, Indianapolis, Indiana

Rebecca Batchelor for her exceptional cover and text design

Carla Hall and all the wonderful staff at the Honor Society of Nursing, Sigma Theta Tau International

Very special thanks to Cindy Saver, who believed in me and was always positive and encouraging in guiding me through the publishing process

And to my dog, Sadie, and my cat, Binky, who lay next to my computer to keep me company during the many hours of writing the book.

Points of Passion Author Notes

While participating in self-care and wellness programs is extremely important to maximize your own health potential, nurses understand better than most people the often-random devastation of disease. A groundbreaking initiative, *The American Center for Cures*, headed by Richard Boxer, MD, and Lou Weisbach, may help change the frustrating, devastating cycle of suffering. To learn more about this initiative, please visit www.theamericancenterforcures.org.

In honor of his mother, a lifelong, passionate knitter, Gary Scholar has published a self empowerment picture book for children titled *Angora: I'm Knot Just Fluff, I'm Always Enough*. As a result of the book, he has created a self empowerment knitting and crocheting initiative for "tween" (8-12 year olds) and teens called "Cast On To Your Dreams." This initiative will be rolled out nationwide by the end of 2010. Besides learning how to knit or crochet, the "Dream Stitchers," as participants are called, will keep journals about their commitment to their dreams, their acts of kindness, and their acceptance of others. One of the objectives of the program is to teach knitting or crocheting to hospitalized children, who may lay in bed for weeks or months at a time, with little constructive to do. This self-empowerment initiative will give sick children something wonderful to occupy their minds, keep their spirits up, and instill pride in their accomplishments.

About the Author

Gary Scholar, M.Ed., is a nationally recognized health and wellness consultant. He spent 10 years as a health and wellness consultant for the employees of the American Hospital Association. He formerly taught at the Department of Health and Research Policy at the University of Illinois, Chicago, on a National Institutes of Health grant, working to lower the severity of multiple chronic illnesses through fitness and health education. He has also contributed numerous wellness articles to the nurse executive magazine *Voice of Nursing Leadership* and to *American Nurse Today*, the official magazine of the American Nurses Association.

Scholar's mission is to be an advocate for nurses and to lead a national call-to-action campaign that benefits the health, wellness, and self-care of nurses everywhere. His immediate goals are to work with hospitals, nursing schools, and communities to create nurse wellness programs, and to initiate a series of wellness awards ceremonies that specifically honor nurses who create healthier lifestyles for themselves. He is available for employee health and wellness consulting, speaking engagements, and book signings. Contact Gary Scholar directly at gscholar@prodigy.net.

Contributing Authors

Karen Redmond

Karen Redmond, MS, is a CHEK-certified CHEK faculty, corrective exercise specialist, and holistic health and lifestyle coach. She has a master's in science in health and fitness promotion and is a master CHEK practitioner and instructor. Karen is the owner of North Shore Smart Bodies in Northbrook, Illinois. She specializes in corrective exercises and holistic lifestyle coaching. She sees a wide variety of clients, including those with orthopedic injuries and back pain. She also works with pre- and post-natal clients and athletes.

Caroline Jung

Caroline Jung, LAc, MSOM, received her undergraduate degree in psychology from the University of Memphis and her master's of science in Oriental medicine from Midwest College of Oriental Medicine. She is a nationally board certified acupuncturist. Jung was part of a pilot program that provided acupuncture and massage for nurses at Children's Memorial Hospital, Chicago Illinois. Jung has been featured in numerous publications including the American Organization of Nurse Executives' journal, *Voice of Nursing Leadership*. Caroline has a special emphasis on treating women's health, digestive disorders, skin disorders, and pain management. She is also a certified yoga teacher.

Raina Childers

Raina Childers, RD, is director of Nutrition Services at Health Point Fitness, a medically integrated fitness center in Cape Girardeau, Missouri. She is a regular on-air face for the CBS affiliate, KFVS 12 (serving southern Illinois, eastern Missouri, western Kentucky, and parts of Tennessee and Arkansas), where she has her own segment called "Cooking With Raina" on the Emmy award winning morning show.

Table of Contents

1   **ICU (Inspired Care for yoU):**
    Starting Your New Lifestyle Shift 1

2   **Assess Yourself:** Giving Yourself the Same
    Honest Assessment You Would Any Patient 13

3   **Take Charge, Nurse:** Assertiveness Training
    for Your Life. 19

4   **Vital Metabolism:** It's Not Just About Waist Sizes 31

5   **In Control:** Managing Blood Pressure, Cholesterol,
    and Blood Sugar 37

6   **How ER (Exercising Regularly) Can Help Keep
    You Out of the ED (Emergency Department)** 47

7   **Taking Back Your Back:** Reducing or Eliminating
    Back Pain Through Fitness 79

8   **Getting Out of Your Comfort Zone:**
    Recognizing the Signs and Changing the
    Behaviors of Comfort Eating 103

9   **Nourish Yourself, Nurse:** Nutrition That Fits
    Your Life 119

10 **When the Night Shift Eclipses You:**
    Special Strategies for Night-Shift Nurses 135

11 **Weighing Your Options:** Weight Management
    for Every Nurse. 147

12 **Holistic Health and Nutrition From Traditional
    Chinese Medicine**. 163

13 **Developing Your Own Life-Support Team** 175

A   **Personalizing Your Assertive Nurse**
     Daily Care Plan 185

B   **Staging Your Own Food Shopping Intervention:**
     Strategies for Navigating Those Dangerous Aisles .193

C   **Recipe RX for RNs** 205

     References 237

     Index 241

Foreword

When I was asked to write a foreword to this book, I was indeed honored, because the topic of fitness in the nursing industry is a great passion of mine. The nursing profession is one of the most honorable professions and offers more opportunities today than ever before. Among the plethora of careers, nursing is a good and noble option; however, with every blessing, there lies a burden. The responsibility, compassion, giving, kindness, and other foundations required for proper patient care also flow into our personal lives and can result in long, tiring days that may deplete our health and interfere with our own self-care.

Gary Scholar, a long-time fitness and wellness guru, became passionate about the health of nurses after he began consulting for the American Hospital Association a number of years ago. What really bothered him, he reports, was that he saw nurses routinely putting others' needs ahead of their own—in all aspects of their lives. While they were constant and effective advocates for their patients, Scholar found it extremely challenging for nurses to convince themselves to make their own needs a priority in their lives. Thus was born his "Nurse Type E Personality" (where nurses do Everything for Everyone but themselves) and his assertive nurse training philosophy.

Each chapter of *Fit Nurse* offers a different aspect of self-care for nurses to consider. The book is full of instruction, solid science, and motivation and inspiration. It also embraces all characteristics of a nurse's life, ranging from back care to food shopping, and leaves no stone unturned, including metabolism, energy, blood values, and night shift challenges. Further, a registered dietitian contributes more than 35 recipes designed to make healthy eating tasty and satisfying.

I will carry this book with me all day, every day, to access the tools Scholar offers. This book, you see, will not weigh more than the baggage we all carry on a daily basis—baggage that proceeds to wear us down, day after day, like a dripping faucet that is never fixed. In my seminar "From Pressure to Peace," a stress management class designed for nurses, I teach participants the importance of balancing mind, body, soul, spirit, home, and work. In this course, each nurse is required to complete a personal health care plan with the same care, love, and devotion they give to each and every one of their patients. I have witnessed how hard this exercise is for nurses to perform, but the teaching tools found in this book walk the reader through the techniques so eloquently that anyone can do it. These step-by-step approaches for making changes disarm the enabled nurse—those type E personality nurses—to be set free and restored to the person that lies within.

I strongly suggest this book to everyone in the medical profession who is passionately committed to shift work, demanding hours, and the loving compassion needed to sustain the fulfillment found in nurse work.

–Judith Henninger, RN, BS, CWC, HLC

Judith Henninger is a registered nurse, a certified corporate wellness coach, and a certified holistic life coach. She works for AtlantiCare's Health Engagement unit in southern New Jersey as a health and wellness educator. AtlantiCare is a recipient of the 2009 Malcolm Baldrige National Quality Award, and its medical center has been designated a nursing Magnet hospital by the American Nurses Credentialing Center.

Introduction

When was the last time you did something really special just for you? If you're like a lot of nurses, the answer might be, "I can't remember!"

I wrote *Fit Nurse: Your Total Plan for Getting Fit and Living Well* with the goal of changing that answer to, "I do something special for myself every day !"

This book will help you rise above the many challenges and struggles you face as a nurse when it comes to your own self-care, fitness, nutrition, weight management, stress management, and well-being. It will provide you with the tools, expertise, and inspiration to transform your lifestyle behaviors for the better.

The inspiration for *Fit Nurse* came from my passionate belief that nurses deserve to be empowered to reconnect with themselves and align their minds and bodies to create healthier lifestyles. The book also evolved from my many years as a health and wellness consultant and passionate nurse advocate. I researched and wrote articles about the disconnect between how much nurses give of themselves to their profession and patients, and how underserved they are when it comes to their own health and well-being.

My priority was to write an empowering wellness book specifically for nurses; I wanted to integrate professional wellness expertise in all area's of a nurse's life and give nurses a voice throughout the book as they talk about their own experiences, challenges, and successes in implementing self-care and creating healthier lifestyles.

The voices of nurses that speak throughout the book were gathered by many interviews I've done with individual nurses across the country and by a survey sent to hundreds of nurses at AtlantiCare Health System in New Jersey.

The five survey questions were

1. As a nurse, what are the challenges that have kept you from pursuing personal self-care and healthier nutrition, regular fitness, or weight management?

2. What do you think is the key trigger that would enable you, as a nurse, to make a paradigm shift and become more proactive in your own self-care and healthier lifestyle?

3. Please explain in detail if you have had success in integrating personal self-care and healthier nutrition, regular fitness, or weight management into your daily life.

4. If you have had success, please write a 2-day food diary and fitness log to show how you have integrated a healthier lifestyle within your hectic, demanding work schedule.

5. Have you ever experienced chronic back pain? If so, how did you treat it?

The book is meant to empower, inspire, and energize all nurses, including hospital nurses, home health nurses, clinical nurses, nurse executives, or school nurses, who struggle with their own self-care and want to shift toward a healthier lifestyle. It is also intended for nurses leading a healthier lifestyle who want more practical knowledge and inspiration. It is especially aimed at students in nursing schools. If you start living well while you're in school, you have a great foundation for continuing a healthier lifestyle by the time you become an RN.

If you are not a nurse but have a friend, co-worker, or family member who is, this book represents the perfect gift for them—the gift of living well!

The book is important to nurses because it provides

- Specific, comprehensive wellness plans that can be successfully integrated on a daily basis, even with your demanding schedule.

- Inspiration on how to raise the quality of your life.

- Professional expertise in numerous areas of your lifestyle, including nutrition, fitness, weight management, and back pain management.

- The energy to be more effective in your job as a nurse.

My hope is that this book represents a bold call to action for all nurses. The big-picture purpose of this book is to create a unified nursing movement with the commitment to change the culture of nursing to place self-care high on the priority list for effective nursing. Ideally, newly graduated nurses can enter a profession that has nurses' best interests at heart.

Thank you so much for the extraordinary opportunity to inspire you to improve your quality of life as a nurse. The positive effects of this improvement are that you are healthier and have more energy to take care of your patients.

RX for Reading the Book

DOSAGE: Read the chapters during daytime or nighttime until completely finished with the book.

REFILLS: You may read the book as many times as you would like, and you may reorder the book for your staff, friends, and colleagues.

DIRECTIONS: Key features of the book:

- Beneficial nutritional and fitness plans, diagrams, and photos are included, designed specifically to empower your self-care.

- *Empowering Nurses* sidebars are positive stories of nurses living the Lifestyle Shift—nurses who are committed to fitness and are examples of success.

- *Livewell* margin notes focus on fitness discussions, definitions, warnings, issues, insights, and so on.

- *Finding Fitness* sidebars are detailed narratives of nurses who have progressed from unfit to fit.

- *Discharge Care Plans* close each chapter by reinforcing key messages of the chapter.

- *I Am at My Best* checklists throughout the book help you feel in control of your health and well-being.

- Appendixes present a daily care plan, a food shopping intervention, and tasty recipes.

INTERACTION: By completing all the interactive portions of a chapter, you will earn a Golden Nightingale Wellness Certificate, which will be awarded to you at the end of Appendix A.

Good luck with your lifestyle shift!

–Gary Scholar, M.Ed.

1

"From this moment on, every voice that told you 'you can't,' is silenced. Every reason that tells you things will never change disappears. The person you were before is over and now it's your turn!"

–From the movie
Freedom Writers
(2007)

ICU (Inspired Care for yoU): Starting Your New Lifestyle Shift

Nurses share a common goal—to make a difference in the lives of patients and clients. This book honors that dedication and challenges you to turn that passion for health and welfare upon yourself, empowering and inspiring you to make a difference in your own life. It gives you a fresh perspective on a more engaged and healthier lifestyle for yourself. You may work the day shift, the night shift, or the rotating shift; you may be a staff nurse, an advanced practice nurse, or an executive nurse; you may be a novice or an expert; yet the most demanding, inspiring, and rewarding shift you will ever work is something I call the *Lifestyle Shift*.

LIVEWELL

Not Funny

Have you heard this one?

A post-surgical cardiac patient is slowly walking down the hospital hall with his physical therapist at his side. The patient notices a very elderly nurse walking toward him.

"What's your secret for a long, healthy, stress-free life?" asks the patient.

"I never exercise. I always eat unhealthy foods in large quantities, and I left my own self care on the delivery table when I was born."

"Wow, that's amazing!" said the patient. "And just how old are you?"

"Twenty-seven," replied the nurse.

Living Well Is the Best Medicine

Many years ago, I attended a nursing conference in my professional role as a health and wellness consultant. There, I spoke with many of the nurses and was surprised at how stressed they appeared and how much they collectively seemed to struggle to maintain a healthy lifestyle. Afterward, I asked myself two questions specific to the nursing profession.

1. Why is it so challenging to implement healthier behaviors for nurses?

2. What can be done to make a paradigm shift so that nurses become more engaged in and protective of their own well-being?

As children, we're regularly asked what we want to be when we grow up. I'm confident that when you pictured yourself as a nurse, you did not visualize a stressed out, unhealthy nurse who is constantly depleted of energy. Unfortunately, because the nursing culture is about extremes—from the long hours to the stress of life-or-death work—many nurses get stuck in destructive self-patterns from the very start of their careers, including the lack of regular physical exercise and using junk food and high-caffeine sodas and coffee as stimulants to keep them alert and functional when they first experience the "culture shock" of full-time nurse work. Once started, these habits and patterns are hard to break.

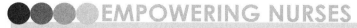

EMPOWERING NURSES

Stop the seesaw, I want to get off!

Karen Hendrickson a bright, charismatic, and successful nurse executive at Southeast Missouri Hospital started asking herself those same critical questions as I asked myself all those years ago—why is it so challenging to implement healthier behaviors for nurses? And what can be done to make a paradigm shift so that nurses become more engaged in and protective of their own well-being?

"I found myself highly educated and successful in my job, but overweight and not as healthy as I wanted to be. I had a hard time making healthy choices and finding the time to exercise, especially when working 12-hour days. The willpower was just not there."

Karen is a perfect example of a nurse performing successfully in her work but underperforming when it comes to her own health and wellness. As is the case with many nurses, this disparity between a successful work life and unsuccessful self care creates a seesaw of unhealthy priorities and unbalanced lifestyle behaviors.

At some point, though, Karen decided to get off the seesaw and get unstuck. The result? She lost 40 pounds, reduced her body mass index (BMI) by 6 points, and dropped 13 inches in her body circumference. While she was at it, she decreased her cholesterol and low-density lipoprotein (LDL). Most importantly, she feels better about herself and has significantly more energy to be engaged both in the work she loves and with her family. Karen's story is one of continuous daily commitment and healthier choices. She does not always find it easy, but it's always rewarding. Karen is not only a success in her work but also in her own self care.

What's her secret? An all-chocolate diet? Chaining herself to her desk so she isn't tempted to inhale the junk food at the nurses' station? Rollerblading down the halls during codes? None of the above: Karen is successfully working her own Lifestyle Shift.

Lifestyle Shift

Working your Lifestyle Shift involves the power of choice. You choose to engage in the process of becoming proactive in your own lifestyle by developing healthier behaviors of nutrition, regular fitness, weight management, and inspired self care. Your results will give you a true sense of fulfillment. You also have a unique opportunity to influence others by becoming a healthier lifestyle role model, potentially inspiring co-workers, friends, and family.

Dr. William Glasser's *Choice Theory* (1998) explains how every behavior you might exhibit is based on your best attempt to meet a need. For you to make the most effective choices, you need to examine and reformulate your thoughts.

The Silent Epidemic

I believe nurses are like master chefs who never get to taste their own exquisite cuisine. You work long hours with incredible attention to detail that makes a difference in the lives of your patients. Yet the opportunity to receive that same exquisite care seldom comes.

●●●●●EMPOWERING NURSES

Silent Epidemic

Remember Karen? She fully understands you cannot create a healthier lifestyle without first acknowledging the elephant in the room—the silent epidemic of nurses denying and disavowing their own self care. Karen acknowledges, "I am a self-confessed 'multitasker' who hardly knows what *relax* means. The stressors in my life both professionally and personally never let up."

As a nurse, you are a director in the theater of health and well-being. In the first act, you advise your patients on the importance of prioritizing self care, healthy nutrition, and regular exercise in their lives. In the second act, you listen to the excuses for why patients don't have time or energy to place self care as a priority (spoiler alert: these are the same reasons you use—hectic schedules and family responsibilities!). In the third act, you watch as the curtain comes down on your patients in the form of devastating chronic lifestyle illnesses such as heart disease, diabetes, obesity, and so on. The playwright in this theater is telling you that it's your turn to be on stage, to put your life, your health, and your wellness in the spotlight.

LIVEWELL

"I believe that nurses tend to take care of everyone else, and then whatever time is left they use it on themselves. I believe we are codependents, and I have found the work of Melody Beattie very helpful. With the help of her book, *Codependent No More* [1992], I started to examine my behaviors more."

–Bonnie, hospice nurse

The great paradox of the nursing profession is that the very function of being the primary caregiver for patients makes it difficult for nurses to implement a healthier lifestyle for themselves. To better understand how to work your Lifestyle Shift, I believe you first need to address the four major challenges (discussed in the next sections of this chapter) that help sabotage your efforts to incorporate a healthier lifestyle.

Nurse Type E Personality

The first major challenge is that most nurses I've encountered have what I call a Nurse Type E personality. What's a Nurse Type E personality? If you are a Nurse Type E personality, you do _everything_ for _everyone_ but yourself, thus denying you of your needs. The Type E personality tends to see self care as either black or white. Either you take care of others, or you are selfish if you take care of yourself.

The Nurse Type E personality has three development stages. I label them the three S's: satisfaction, significance, and sacrifice.

The first stage of development for the Nurse Type E personality begins when you are a child. As a child, you exhibit a very nurturing heart, and you learn by giving comfort to others that you always receive inner _satisfaction_, for example, the satisfaction of being there for a friend who has gone through a challenging life episode.

The second development stage occurs when you receive positive encouragement for your compassionate ability to take care of others' needs. This encouragement makes you feel _significant_. For example, you might volunteer at a homeless or pet shelter, and your parents then tell you how proud they are of you.

"Part of proper self care is identifying what you are feeling."

The third development stage for your Nurse Type E personality is the big payoff. You actually get _paid_ to be a Type E personality when you become a nurse. In your job, you are encouraged to _sacrifice_ for the needs of others. Being put in this position is comparable to being a diabetic chocoholic in the role of chief executive of a chocolate factory. With long-practiced ease, you sacrifice your needs to the doctors, patients, and your own family and friends.

As a result of the three development stages of the Nurse Type E personality, you might feel deep inside that you don't deserve care for yourself. This attitude is a reflection of how you see yourself. For example, "I'm too tired after taking care of everyone and everything to exercise." What you are really saying to yourself is that you don't deserve to feel healthier, be better physically and emotionally, or to have more energy through the benefits of exercise. When you perceive that you have a low "deserve" level, it corresponds directly to higher stress, depleted energy, and burnout.

Imagine if you were encouraged, since you were young, to make it a priority to place self care into your daily life. How would that have changed your lifestyle behaviors and the nursing profession?

Proper self care is identifying what you are feeling. Please answer these three questions that can help with your own self-awareness. You can ask yourself these questions any time you feel overwhelmed.

1. Why do I feel drained?

2. What do I need at this moment?

3. Where do I need to create healthier boundaries in my life?

LIVEWELL

"For 22 years, I worked as a staff nurse on mostly 12-hour shifts, but 12 hours often turned into 14 hours. By the time I got home, I was exhausted, starved, thirsty, and stressed out. After I got home, I still had to raise my two beautiful children and take them to ballet lessons, soccer, guitar lessons, church activities, basketball, tennis, and softball. Who has the time or energy to think about taking care of yourself?"

–Ginger, clinical educator

Some nurses experience compassion fatigue, which is overcare to the point of burnout. In her groundbreaking book *The Wisdom of Menopause* (2006, p. 86-87) author Christiane Northrup talks about self-sacrifice, "The more honest we are with ourselves about the motivation that drives our choices, the healthier we will be. This is as true for caregiving as it is for any other area of our lives, perhaps even more so." She goes on and talks about care and overcare. "True care of others, from a place of unconditional love, enhances our health. But overcare and burnout destroy our health and run our batteries down. Overcare is often motivated by guilt and unfinished business, for which we hope to somehow compensate through the caregiving role" (2006, p. 86-87)

In her book, *The Art of Extreme Self-Care* (2009, p. 4), Cheryl Richardson wrote, "I've come to learn that overgiving is often a sign of deprivation—a signal that a need isn't being met, an emotion isn't being expressed, or a void isn't getting filled. Becoming aware of how and why you feel deprived can be a key to recognizing what needs to shift emotionally and physically to achieve extreme self care."

Shift Work—Second Shift Syndrome

The second major challenge facing nurses to integrate healthier lifestyles is shift work and long working hours. Shift work can exacerbate poor self care habits because of the long, demanding, stressful hours that a nurse works, leaving little time and energy to focus on a nurse's own needs. Rotating shifts can make it challenging to implement a regularly scheduled self care plan on a daily basis. Night shifts can take a huge toll on a nurse's health and well-being by throwing the circadian rhythm out of sync, causing sleep disturbances and making it extremely challenging to integrate self care, healthy eating, and regular exercise on a daily basis. The nurses in the Empowering Nurses sidebar clearly illustrate that your overwhelming responsibility as a nurse doesn't stop at the door when you get home. This situation is referred to as the Second Shift Syndrome.

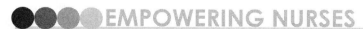 EMPOWERING NURSES

Raising the Red Flag

A nurse would go home after a long 12-hour shift at the hospital and immediately start taking care of the needs of her family—making dinner, cleaning the house, helping the kids with homework, giving support to her husband's issues at work, and so on.

The nurse realized she never had time to decelerate from her job and to shift gears before being plunged into her family's needs. She felt completely depleted of energy and felt severe burnout.

The nurse explained her situation to a neighbor who happened to be a wellness coach. The coach gave her the advice to wear a red scarf when she got home everyday as a signal to her family to give her time and space to wind down. Then, once she took off the scarf, she would be available for her family.

When her neighbor checked in a few weeks later, she told him "It really works! So my husband went out and bought a red tie!"

LIVEWELL

"I think one of the biggest obstacles in maintaining a healthier lifestyle for a nurse is the long and varied shifts. I'm amazed that anyone would want to work a 12-hour shift—which is more like 13 or 14 hours—and then have the energy to go to the gym. I work nights. This is bound to affect your health and overall energy level. It can cause nurses to eat poorly on top of everything else. Then you have the varied shifts. You work days and nights. Sometimes that means working all 12-hour shifts (a.m. or p.m.) or 12's and 8's at any given time. It takes a huge toll on your body. The body has no consistency. Nurses who are mothers and work nights have an increasing demand. They might work all night and then get home and get the kids off to school, not getting themselves into bed until after 9:00 a.m. Then if they have to pick the kids up again around 3:00 p.m., they have to be up at 2:30 p.m. It's just not enough sleep. Or if they work a weekend night, they might have to be at the soccer game or birthday party."

—Lauren, traveling pediatric ICU nurse

Food

The third major challenge you might face in integrating a healthier lifestyle is inconsistent eating. When the body receives nourishing sources of nutrition, all of our body systems operate at an optimal level. Nutritious food is supportive of overall balance and good energy.

There are many challenges and struggles that nurses confront when trying to eat healthier. Temptation is everywhere: There's the unhealthy thank-you gifts patients' families bring in and the junk food snacking at vending machines, nurses' stations, and break rooms because you don't have the time to eat breakfast, lunch, or dinner. Sitting down to eat? A horse sits more than a nurse does! Factor in the "dumping" of junk food on co-workers (because you don't want your family to eat all that junk!) and celebrating every birthday and holiday on the calendar (and some that are made up!) with unhealthy comfort food, and you have the prescription for any number of physical and mental conditions.

●●●●●EMPOWERING NURSES

In the Night Kitchen

"Working night shifts has negatively impacted my eating habits," reports Lauren. "I can say personally that I have gotten up at 2 a.m. on a night when I'm not working to eat. On most units there is *always* food around. I find that parents bring the staff food as an offering of gratitude, and it's typically cookies, candies, cake, cupcakes, and other junk foods. We just eat and eat. It's also a pretty well-known fact that if you have food in your house that you don't want to consume yourself, just bring it to the break room at the hospital. It will be gone in a flash. This happens all the time! Our unit has potluck lunches all the time. It's always a nurse's last shift or birthday or baby shower or bridal shower—any reason to bring in food and eat. For example, this week my unit is having a Mardi Gras potluck."

Stress

The fourth major challenge you might face is stress. As a nurse you could feel stressed out because of the challenges you face, including:

- An overload of patients

- Floating to different floors

- Rotating shifts, night shifts, and long hours

- Conflict with doctors

- Dealing with difficult family members

- Coping with the emotional toll of losing a patient

- Patient care issues

- Uncertainty concerning treatment

- Concerns of technical knowledge and skills

- Overtime, endless paper work

- Sleep issues

- Working a second or third job

New nurses might feel overwhelmed with responsibility. Nurse executives might have to deal with staff shortages, morale issues, retention and recruitment, quality of care for patients, budget constraints, lack of time, and so on. This doesn't even include the stress caused by your personal life. (I got exhausted just typing the list.) You face this stress endlessly on a daily basis. The result is that nurses suffer from an energy crisis and are at huge risk for burnout.

LIVEWELL

For Whom the Stress Tolls

"Orders are coming from residents, ARNPs, and PAs, and many of them will be changed by attending physicians. Meanwhile the nurse is the one running around making phone calls to clarify orders. Calls from different departments follow up to complete ordered tests, labs, consults, medication orders, therapies, and so on, and again the nurse has to know how to juggle and prioritize the plan of care, must know how many patients they are responsible for, must keep patients safe, must medicate on time, and must have them ready to be taken away by different department/therapies so that orders can be completed. Stress? You also have to be ready to deal with an emergency such as a fall or a code or be ready to offer emotional support to patients and families who have received bad news. And don't forget getting patients ready to be discharged. Everyone wants to leave first! And then come the admissions in the middle of all the chaos!"

–Carmen, clinical and hospital nurse

Working It

So how do you rise above all your difficult challenges and implement a healthier lifestyle? The answer is you can empower yourself by working your Lifestyle Shift. A Lifestyle Shift is a paradigm shift toward implementing healthier nutrition, regular fitness, weight management, and inspiring self care.

It's easier to stay in your comfort zone, even when it doesn't fit your needs, because it takes less effort than the energy required to make a change. That's why you need to make a compelling case for yourself to make a shift out of your comfort zone.

As a nurse, you have your own personal reasons to make the shift. It might be a last straw event because of your health. Or you might make the change because of your depleted energy and elevated stress level. Or maybe it's just to maintain your current wellness level. There are a number of reasons that might incite you to make a change. The important thing is that it's your reason.

LIVEWELL

Shifting

"I've matured enough to know that I cannot do everything I want to do, but if I want to be healthier and enjoy my children and grandchildren, healthy nutrition and exercise are the key for me, just like I've been telling my patients all these years. I've quit smoking. I've been going to the health club 3 days a week. I've lost 13 pounds, with only 9 more pounds to reach my goal. This all requires planning— planning for time, grocery shopping, menus, and so on. I would like to think that I could have done it sooner. I'm just happy to finally be getting there now!"

–Ginger

Florence Nightingale (1859) wrote, "What nurses have to do is to put the patient in the best condition for nature to act upon them." I believe that statement can be flipped; as a nurse, you need to put yourself in the best possible condition to promote your own healthier lifestyle.

Whatever your catalyst is to make the shift, I'm just proud of you to be taking the first steps by reading this book. It's never too late to make a difference in your own life!

In the following chapters you are going to learn proactive steps to live a more balanced, healthier, and more connected lifestyle. I am going to be with you every step of the way, encouraging and supporting your efforts to work your Lifestyle Shift. This is your new call to action and mission of service. *It's all about you.* You deserve it, and I know you can do it.

Discharge Care Plan

In your work as a nurse, you have to constantly prioritize. Just for fun, to be formally discharged from this chapter, please use your prioritizing nursing skill to reinforce some of the key messages of the chapter. Prioritize the following in order of importance, with 1 being the most important, and 3 being the least important. Answers are at the bottom of the page, upside down.

A. __ Nurse Type E personality has three stages of development: satisfaction, significant, and sacrifice.

B. __ Identifying your Nurse Type E personality, food, stress, and shift work as challenges in creating a healthier lifestyle helps give you clarity of what you need to overcome.

C. __ Creating a healthier lifestyle is a power of choice.

D. __ Some nurses have a Type M & M's personality. Just give them an IV of chocolate, and they'll be happy.

Congratulations! You have earned a Golden Nightingale Wellness Wing for completing the interactive portion of this chapter. The goal is to earn all 13 Wings to be awarded your Golden Nightingale Wellness Wing certificate at the end of Appedix A.

(A = 3; B = 2; C = 1; D = 4)

2

"My current lifestyle was created by choices I made yesterday. My optimal lifestyle is the power of my choices starting today."

–Gary Scholar

Lifestyle Assessment: Giving Yourself the Same Honest Assessment You Would Any Patient

Why do some nurses succeed in creating healthier lifestyles while others struggle to even start the process? What is the tipping point that propels some nurses forward into positive lifestyle changes while others are left behind with deepened feelings of failure?

After looking at all the many responses I received during the development of this book, I've found two main tipping points for those who charged forward in their Lifestyle Shift.

1. The concern for health: weight gain, high blood pressure, cholesterol, pre-diabetes or diabetes, and so on.

2. The age of offspring, if there were any. Nurses with children who have left home were more likely to focus on themselves.

LIVEWELL

In Perspective

The difference between not living well and living well is the difference between watching your dirty bathtub water trickle down a stuck drain or standing before a magnificent ocean vista. The first is draining; the second is empowering!

"What's missing from your lifestyle is the integration of high-performance re-energizing ingredients of inspiring self care that honors the best of who you are and includes a dash of healthier nutrition and regular fitness that won't weigh you down."

One of my hopes in writing this book is to have nurses create healthier lifestyles before they find themselves with health concerns or to have them avoid waiting so many years to finally take care of themselves. Children can and should be taught to respect their parents' need for self care; otherwise we just continue to perpetuate the destructive cycles in the next generation.

To have success in creating a healthier lifestyle, you might need to change your current lifestyle by transforming the daily choices you make in order to integrate what's really important to you, in other words, to give yourself a clear and honest picture of what is really worth your energy and focus given your extreme time constraints as a nurse. The more energy and focus you give to integrating what's important to you, the greater your health and well-being rewards.

To give you clarity in your pursuit of working your Lifestyle Shift, you need to first examine your current lifestyle and how you want to transform it. A good strategy to create a visual picture of your current lifestyle is to visualize your lifestyle as a food plate.

As a nurse, you tend to have a lot dumped on your plate. Your full plate contains a heavy amount of long, saturated hours full of stressful responsibilities peppered with personal responsibilities. Top this with a calorie-laden sauce of competing role expectations as a nurse, parent, spouse/partner, friend, community service leader, and so on, and daily consumption of your current lifestyle can deplete you of your energy and passion, causing you to feel totally overwhelmed. You can lose who you really are with your unhealthy, laden, king-sized portioned lifestyle.

What's missing from your lifestyle is the integration of high-performance re-energizing ingredients of inspiring self care that honors the best of who you are and includes a dash of healthier nutrition and regular fitness that won't weigh you down.

To begin working your Lifestyle Shift, you measure your current lifestyle against your optimal lifestyle. The difference can give you clarity by showing you what you need to focus on as you work your Lifestyle Shift. The portions on your plate, the areas of your life that you need to examine and measure, consist of the following:

- Job
- Personal responsibilities
- Self care, for example, time you spend pursuing a hobby, to have massage, to read a book, and so on.
- Healthier nutrition
- Regular fitness

Because nurses experience extreme daily time constraints, you need to measure your focus, effort, and energy you apply to each portion of your lifestyle plate per day instead of the time you put in. Joan is a 43 year old RN on a hospital cancer floor, who works the day shift. She is married with 3 children ages 15, 12, and 7 years old. Joan feels she has no time or energy for her own self care, including her hobbies of reading, knitting, gardening and playing tennis—which she hasn't done for many years. She is overweight, has Type 2 diabetes, and does not exercise. Her demanding schedule and responsibilities have created a lot of stress which she copes with by unhealthy comfort eating. Joan is burned out.

For example, Joan's current daily lifestyle plate consists of her job and her personal responsibilities.

Joan's Current Lifestyle

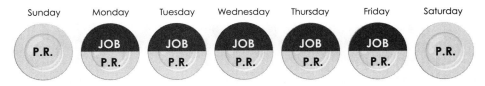

P.R. = Personal Responsibilities

Joan wants her optimal daily lifestyle plate to reflect what she really believes will meet her needs. She would love to strive for a healthier lifestyle that gives her a soft place to land everyday for her own personal self care. Joan would like to schedule in tennis twice a week and walk 3 other days for 40 minutes. She would also want to schedule in preparing healthy meals on Sundays to take to work during the week. This would allow her not to be tempted at work with all the junk food. She would also want to schedule in reading, knitting, or gardening at least twice a week. Joan feels that by taking care of her needs it will help her become healthier and lose some weight. It would also help empower and reenergize herself so she would be a happier and more effective nurse, mother, and a better partner to her husband.

Joan's Optimal Lifestyle

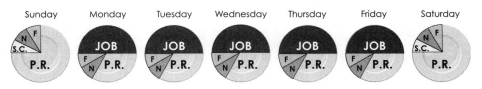

P.R. = Personal Responsibilities   **N** = Nutrition Healthy   **S.C.** = Self Care   **F** = Fitness

Now it's your turn. Fill in your lifestyle plates and answer the following questions. Please be honest with yourself.

Your Current Lifestyle

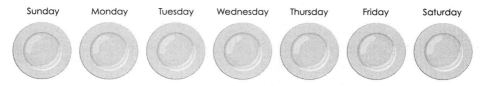

P.R. = Personal Responsibilities   N = Nutrition Healthy   S.C. = Self Care   F = Fitness

Evaluating Your Current Lifestyle

1. After reviewing your lifestyle plates, are you satisfied with your current lifestyle?

2. Would you recommend your current lifestyle to your patients, family, children, or friends?

3. What problematic patterns do you see emerging from your current lifestyle?

Your Optimal Lifestyle

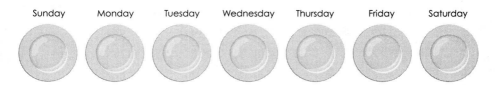

P.R. = Personal Responsibilities   N = Nutrition Healthy   S.C. = Self Care   F = Fitness

Charting Your Goals

I am at my best when: For example, you feel either empowered, fulfilled, reenergized, or using your full potential when engaged in a specific activity or trying to attain a goal.

1. What specific self care goals would you like to integrate into your lifestyle? I am at my best when: For example, engaged in knitting an afghan blanket, scheduling a massage, or gardening.

2. What specific healthier nutrition goals would you like to integrate into your lifestyle? I am at my best when: For example, I eat a healthy breakfast every day, cut out sodas and replace them with water, and read food labels that restrict my sugar intake to 6 grams or less per serving.

3. What specific regular fitness goals would you like to integrate into your lifestyle? I am at my best when: For example, weight training for 30 minutes 3 days a week, 40 minutes of yoga 2 times a week, and playing volleyball once a week.

The great thing about using the visualization technique of the food plate is that it effortlessly helps to reinforce your focus on working your Lifestyle Shift. Every time you look at a plate of food it can be a reminder of your lifestyle goals. I'm confident that when you decide to make the effort to create a healthier lifestyle, you are going to succeed! Realistic sustained effort is the true measure of success.

Discharge Care Plan

To be formally discharged from this chapter, please use your nursing prioritization skills to reinforce some of the key messages of the chapter. Place what you think would be the correct prioritized number 1-4 in order of importance next to the corresponding letter.

A. __ Your current lifestyle might drain you of your energy, health, and well-being.

B. __ Examining your current lifestyle against your optimal lifestyle gives you clarity concerning what is really important to you and what your future goals are.

C. __ Every time you look at a plate of food it serves as a reminder of where you need to place your focus, effort, and energy to attain a healthier lifestyle.

D. __ Optimal lifestyle is watching your spouse do all the housework and cooking for the rest of your life.

Congratulations! You have earned a Golden Nightingale Wellness Wing by completing the interactive portions of the chapter!

(A = 2; B = 1; C = 3; D = 4)

"If I am just surviving,
I am settling for less than I
truly deserve."

–Gary Scholar

Take Charge, Nurse:
Assertiveness Training for Your Long Run

If you feel constantly overwhelmed, the result is you do not have the time or the energy for your own self care, which can ultimately take a significant toll on your health and well-being. You might also be subject to negative effects on your sleep, which contributes to weight gain, food cravings, and a weakened immune system.

Of all the feedback I received from nurses during the development of this book, consider the number one challenge to building a healthier lifestyle—feeling completely overwhelmed.

Assert Yourself

Nurses, nor anyone else, should settle for living an overwhelmed life. You deserve a lifestyle that honors and serves your best interests. Fortunately, those panicky feelings of being overwhelmed can be reversed to allow for peace and calm when you become more proactive on your own behalf.

The most effective strategy to overcome feeling overwhelmed is to integrate one of your most powerful leadership strengths currently used in your role as a nurse—assertiveness.

As a nurse, you have the amazing capacity to prioritize and make assertive decisions regarding your patients. However, even though in your work you might be assertive and overperform, you might be more passive and underperform when it comes to your own personal self care.

Assertiveness helps you clearly see the possibilities when it comes to your own care. Assertiveness empowers you by helping you be proactive for your own best interest. You become what you believe by the powerful choices you make.

LIVEWELL

Where Does the Energy Go?

"I feel constantly overwhelmed because I lack the time and energy to manage both my home and full-time work!"

–Pam, hospital RN

When it comes to being assertive, complete the following statement: "I am at my best when I _____ (fill in the blank)" By completing the following statement it will emphasize the importance to be assertive which will make you feel either empowered, reenergized, or fulfilled. It will also identify specific areas that you would like to be more assertive in which would lead to a positive impact on your health and well-being.

Another way to recognize and build your assertiveness is to ask yourself the following question: What are the three proudest accomplishments I have had in my career as a nurse?

Consider the characteristics, the personality traits, that each of these proud moments required from you. Assertiveness is likely one of the key traits for success in each of the three cases. This is because it empowered you to attain a goal, take control of a situation, or make a difference. Assertiveness can play a role in ways you may not be aware of. For example, modeling assertiveness for others may enhance their lives, including the role modeling of strong behaviors for your children who see through the eyes of their parents what they need to learn. Assertiveness can also enhance a relationship by creating open communication when you place your needs on the table. It can also positively impact your health and well-being by making sure your needs are at the top of your priority list. So now you need to use that great strength of yours for your own assertive self care training.

Belief in Self

The key to implementing assertiveness, I believe, stems from a belief in yourself. Even if you feel confident in making life or death decisions with your patients, you may still struggle with believing in yourself outside of work. I know many nurses who are frustrated by trying to keep the weight off, trying to sustain physical activity, or trying to eat healthier. And because staying healthy is so challenging for nurses in the work environment, they lose the belief and trust in themselves to succeed to create that healthier lifestyle.

However, success breeds success! By practicing assertiveness, you can claim small, consistent victories, which can raise your belief and trust in yourself that you can succeed in creating a healthier lifestyle. For example, not skipping breakfast every morning can lead to a healthier blood sugar level and effective weight management and increased energy. Or waking up and performing 5 minutes of safe and effective back exercises can help strengthen your core muscles and help manage your chronic back pain.

Assertiveness and Codependency

Your heart works nonstop just like you do. It delivers blood to every part of your body, but your heart's first priority is to be assertive and take care of number one first. Your heart is not a Type E personality, nor is it codependent. It provides blood first to itself; then it provides the blood needed for the rest of your body. You, too, can learn this lesson from your own anatomy! You have to take care of yourself first before you can successfully take care of others. Codependency in this context is the attempt to meet others' needs to the point of neglecting yourself. The lesson to be learned is that even your own organs understand that the greatest gift you can give yourself is the importance of nurturing your own well-being, which also helps define who you really are and what's important to you.

LIVEWELL

Codependent No More

"I have been an RN for 30 plus years and just thought caring about others was my purpose on Earth. It took some time, but I learned to become assertive and take care of myself first. This includes physically, emotionally, and spiritually. Unless I take care of myself, I really cannot be there for others. I can slip into old patterns and put others' needs before mine, although I am more aware when I do that. My journey has been one of getting to know myself and learning what I need, want, and enjoy. I continue to explore and get to know my likes and dislikes. Some of the things that I do [to stay healthy] include meditation, yoga, and regular exercise. I also eat healthy and drink plenty of water. I rest when I'm tired and sleep longer if I need to. I have healthy people in my life and people who support me on my journey. I work on having balance between work and play in my life. I'm a work in progress because I have had more years taking care of others than I do of taking care of myself."

–Bonnie, hospice nurse

Job Performance

What if your nurse executive or manager sat you down and announced a new job performance review system that included 360 degree feedback? 360 degree feedback is a job review process that involves both your boss and your co-workers. And what if, additionally, 50% of your job performance as a nurse suddenly depended on how well you integrate your assertiveness for your own self care?

Your 360 degree, 50% job performance review consists of the following:

- Display assertiveness for getting your needs met.

- Build trust with yourself in following through with your commitments of self care.

- Focus on achieving your self care goals.

- Inspire positive energy in yourself that sustains change.

- Model transformational self care Lifestyle Shifts to your staff and family.

- Champion self growth through integrating self care.

If you faced this job performance review, how would you approach your job differently? How would you fulfill and schedule in your job performance goals for your own self care on a daily basis?

For some nurses, becoming more assertive is difficult. Even the most successful nurses who apply assertiveness on behalf of their own self care have failed numerous times. That's because persistence and commitment are the keys to learning how to be more assertive. If you continuously practice those two key elements, they increase your ability to make a shift toward sustained change.

Please write a letter to yourself explaining why you deserve to be assertive in creating a healthier lifestyle? One of the major factors for nurses not to implement assertiveness is because they truly feel they don't deserve to get their needs met. By answering the question it will give yourself permission to get your needs met.

Looping

It's time to look at applying assertiveness in helping you manage your daily stress and your feelings of being overwhelmed. I want to first examine what I call *looping*. Looping is when you can't stop worrying about something, and you loop it over and over again in your mind causing you added stress.

Everyone loops at one time or another. When you constantly feel stressed and overwhelmed, looping raises its ugly head. You end up giving away all your precious energy and placing it in the negative spin cycle of looping. Some nurses experience looping right before they go to bed. They end up having difficulty falling asleep, or they wake up during sleep and start looping. This cycle creates sleep deprivation for a nurse who already might be sleep deprived. What your mind obsesses, your body expresses.

Identify your own experiences of looping so you can change detrimental behavior. For your own best interest please be specific in answering the following questions:

- Have you ever experienced looping relating to your job? What did you loop about?

- Have you ever experienced looping in your personal life? What did you loop about?

- Have you ever experienced looping when it came to your weight because your clothes didn't fit?

- Have you ever experienced looping because you beat yourself up regarding eating junk food or not exercising regularly?

- Have you ever experienced looping because of poor body image?

Assertive Steps

Implementing assertiveness helps stop you from looping. As a highly educated nurse, you are no doubt aware that your brain is divided into two hemispheres. (No, one hemisphere is not for chocolates and the other for chocolate chip ice cream.) Your right brain is the center for emotion, and the left brain is the center for reasoning. Looping happens when you have a conflict between the two. For example, what do you feel when you eat a large portion of unhealthy junk food?

Your right brain feels guilty and distressed. Your left brain tells you to eat healthier.

Four assertive steps can help stop your looping.

1. Identify your looping: For example, eating large quantities of unhealthy food, causing weight gain.

2. Identify what you need: For example, to eat healthier.

3. Articulate why you need it: For example, to fit into the clothes you want to wear and improve your body image, health, and energy.

4. Take assertive action: You will let go of beating yourself up. You will empower yourself by limiting the temptation by getting rid of unhealthy foods in your kitchen.

This assertive process lets you step back from looping and view it from a different perspective.

Because we are being honest here I can admit that I have looped about writing this book. So I implemented the four assertive steps:

1. Identify my looping: Writing this book.

2. Identify what I need: To empower and give useful insight for nurses to create healthier lifestyles.

3. Articulate why I need it: Not to disappoint a group of professionals that I have the highest respect for because they make an enormous difference in the lives of millions of patients.

4. Take assertive action: Place my own personality, creativeness, passion, and encouragement into every page I write.

Some effective ways to implement the four assertive steps are taking a clarity walking break for a few minutes, writing in a journal before you fall asleep, and talking out your looping to someone who is supportive.

> "Setting healthy boundaries gives you clarity to make empowered choices of what you will and will not do based on your own best interests."

Assertive Boundary Setting

I often ask nurses how they are doing. The typical response is "I'm fine." Well, fine is spelled F-I-N-E. I think it stands for Frequently Ignoring Needs and Emotions. I also hear from nurses that they feel guilty if they aren't taking care of everyone. Guilt is spelled G-U-I-L-T, and I think it stands for Guaranteeing You Infinite Lifetime Therapy!

Part of feeling guilty and ignoring your needs comes from not wanting to disappoint others' expectations—expectations that play heavily into your nurse Type E personality.

An integral skill of assertiveness is how to set healthy boundaries in your pursuit of creating a healthier lifestyle. Setting healthy boundaries gives you clarity to make empowered choices of what you will and will not do based on your own best interests. It honors who you really are. It also challenges and shifts your tendencies away from being a Type E personality.

Like many nurses, you multitask so much that it drastically raises your stress level and your feelings of being overwhelmed, giving you a constant need to set boundaries. Sometimes you have to force yourself to step out of your comfort zone to define where that boundary needs to be. An uncomfortable boundary might be wanting to confront (I prefer *"express your needs"*) your charge nurse to ask for a different shift or more days off because you're feeling burned out. However, you don't want to burden your charge nurse—because the department is short staffed anyway—so actually expressing your needs to your charge nurse makes you feel uncomfortable. Getting past that discomfort and actually talking with your charge nurse to redefine your boundaries will both free and empower you. It's always your right to redefine your needs and boundaries.

What I have found over and over is that when you do become more comfortable applying assertive healthy boundary setting, the people who you're afraid to disappoint end up respecting you more.

●●●● EMPOWERING NURSES

Your Assertiveness Training Lifestyle Shift

Raina Childers, a colleague of mine and a registered dietician and director of nutrition services at Healthpoint Fitness, uses assertiveness training and healthy boundary setting in her work with many of her nurse clients. Raina explains, "I have found that nurses have a difficult time being assertive when it comes to their own health. I work on assertiveness training and the setting of healthy boundaries to help the nurses move their own health up on the priority list of their lives. I like to challenge them with the line, 'If you are not taking care of yourself, what are you doing that is more important?'

"I try to teach nurses to ask the right questions, make the right decisions, and retake control of their lives. I role play with them. We practice conversations. They might practice talking to a waitress, making special requests for their food preparation, or they might try to talk differently to an unsupportive friend or relative who continually sabotages their efforts. They share with me what they admire most about people they describe as 'assertive.' I have them describe how they perceive certain circumstances would be different for them if they communicated assertively as well.

"Setting healthy boundaries might mean that he or she won't eat at buffets anymore because of difficulty in that environment. It might mean that if he or she is asked to work late on a day or evening with an existing personal appointment (a planned workout, a massage, or simply are looking forward to cooking a healthy dinner), he or she says, 'I'm sorry, I can't work late today, but I would be glad to do so another day this week.' A boundary has been set.

"I think the most important thing I focus on with my nursing clients is that to be assertive and to change, one must patiently and persistently accept that this is truly a process. We are all part of a culture that encourages us to become impatient when change is not immediate or easy. Staying the course can be frustrating at times, and I continually remind them of how exceptional they are when they push through to be assertive and create healthy boundaries for themselves."

It's important for co-workers, families, and friends to understand you are fully committed to creating a healthier lifestyle. As a nurse you might feel uncomfortable asking for help, but you need to identify and ask for resources outside yourself. Healthy boundary setting might include having your spouse/partner assume more household responsibilities. Nurses so often enable their spouse/partner because they are Type E personality and try to do everything for their family. It's time to ask for help doing the housework, cooking, or taking care of the children. It's time to give back to you!

Assertiveness Training Examples

Making a special request to a waitress/waiter: How is the food prepared? Is it possible to have the dressing and sauces on the side?

Nurses station or break room—"One more bite won't hurt you!": Would you please not offer me the food? I'm working on trying to be healthier. I would really appreciate it if we could designate a drawer or cabinet for the unhealthy snack foods so I won't be tempted.

Spouse/partner sharing more of the responsibilities at home: If we could designate a time in the morning when you are in charge of the children so I can get my exercise/meditation in, I would really appreciate it because I'm trying very hard to be as healthy and to help manage my stress level as I can.

Deadline at work interfering with a fitness training session or massage, etc.: Is it possible that we could change the time line when this report needs to be completed? I would really appreciate it for I have a prior commitment.

Fitness: I will honor my need for physical activity by scheduling in fitness on _____ days.

Nutrition: I will honor my need to eat healthier by taking the time to make a healthy lunch to bring to work.

- Define what assertiveness looks like to you.
- Define what nonassertiveness looks like to you.

Use self dialog when it comes to your body image and comfort eating, reminding yourself how multidimensional you are: What do you like about yourself that has nothing to do with your physical looks? What makes you happy besides anything food-related?

In the following chapters you are going to apply your assertiveness training as a Take Charge Nurse to empower you to take action.

Discharge Care Plan

You are already exceptional. When you add assertive self care, you feel so much more in control of your life, and you will feel extremely proud of yourself. I know I'm proud of you for taking this important step.

Looking for your discharge papers from this chapter? Please use your nurse prioritizing skills to reinforce some of the key messages discussed throughout this chapter. Place what you think are the correct prioritized number 1-6 in importance next to the corresponding letter.

A. __ Integrating assertiveness for your own self care empowers you to be proactive for your own best interest.

B. __ Use the four assertive steps to help manage your looping.

    1. Identify your looping.

    2. Identify what you need.

    3. Articulate why you need it.

    4. Take assertive action.

C. __ Assertive healthy boundary setting gets your needs met.

D. __ Self care assertiveness is best served when you:

1. Display assertiveness for getting your needs met.

2. Build trust with yourself in following through with your commitments of self care.

3. Focus on achieving your self care goals.

4. Inspire self for positive energy that sustains change.

5. Model a transformational self care Lifestyle Shift to your staff and family.

6. Champion self growth through integrating self care.

E. __ Belief in yourself is key to implementing assertiveness.

F. __ Getting my needs met means scheduling an hour massage before, during, and after each one of my shifts.

Congrats! You have earned a Golden Nightingale Wellness Wing by completing the interactive portions of the chapter!

(A = 1; B = 4; C = 5; D = 3; E = 2; F = 6)

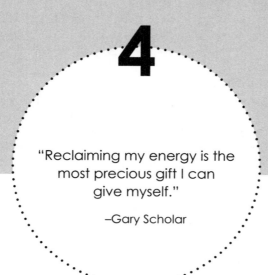

4

"Reclaiming my energy is the most precious gift I can give myself."

–Gary Scholar

Vital Metabolism:
It's Not Just About Waist Sizes

Metabolism, schmetabolism! Why is it so important for you as a nurse to focus on your metabolism? Your long stressful working hours, rotating or night shifts, lack of proper sleep, skipped meals, unhealthy eating patterns, and lack of daily fitness can all contribute to a compromised metabolism that was meant to keep you healthy and energized.

Think of your metabolism as your patient. If you provide your patient with the correct treatment plan, your patient's energy level, health, and well-being drastically improve. But if you don't provide proper care—an IV for nutrition, daily physical therapy, and proper sleep—your patient can end up in the intensive care unit.

LIVEWELL

Metabolism Defined

Your metabolism is biochemistry involving your hormones and enzymes. It transforms the food you eat into the energy your body requires and also affects how well you burn that energy as calories. A functional metabolism keeps your hormones balanced and helps with your weight management.

Table 4.1 provides a blueprint of how your metabolism expends energy. This information is significant because it shows that you have a certain amount of control in raising your own metabolism through eating smaller meals throughout the day and placing fitness into your daily life.

Table 4.1   Energy Expenditure

Percentage of your total calories burned:

60-70%	Your basal metabolic rate (BMR) represents the calories expended to keep your body functioning even at rest.
10%	Thermic effect of food (TEF) represents the calories expended every time you eat.
Up to 30%	Physical activity energy expenditure (PAEE) is what I call the x factor because it is dependent on the amount and intensity of your physical activity.

Your metabolism can also be affected by your:

Age	Metabolism can slow to about 5% per decade after 40 years old. Hey, isn't that age discrimination? Of course, if you're like me, you'll always be 39 years old!
Body Composition	Men tend to lose weight faster because they tend to have more lean muscle than women have. Lean muscle has a higher rate of calories burned at rest than fat has.

Stress

Managing daily stress is one of the challenges nurses face. Chronic stress stimulates the release of the hormone cortisol. An article in the February, 2008, issue of *Prevention* magazine titled "Outsmart Your Cravings," Sally Kuzemchak,

RD, quoted experts stating, "This signals your brain to seek out rewards. Comfort foods loaded with sugar and fat basically blunt this hormone. The food gets coded in your memory center as a solution to unpleasant experience or emotion."

For nurses the release of cortisol can be associated with overeating and craving high-calorie fatty and sugary foods at your nurse's stations or at home.

Due to a nurses demanding work and schedule toxic stress can occur. To help cope with the toxic stress many nurses turn to unhealthy comfort eating which can trigger weight gain.

In her book, *The Wisdom of Menopause*, Christine Northrup, M.D., (2006) writes about the connection between toxic stress and toxic weight gain: "Dr. Pamela Peek, in her book *Fight Fat After Forty*, explains toxic weight gain—the kind of weight that accumulates in the abdomen. She explains about toxic stress coming from resurfacing of childhood trauma, perfectionism, and relationship changes such as divorce and care giving, job stress, acute or chronic illness, dieting and the effects of menopause."

Weight Management

Many nurses have written me about the frequency of skipped meals because of the lack of time in their daily schedules. If every nurse contributed a dime every time he or she skipped a meal, we could create a nursing fund that would pay for stressed out nurses to vacation in Maui at a five-star spa for a month every year.

When you skip a breakfast, lunch, or dinner or wait too long between meals, it slows down your metabolism. It triggers your body to say, "I have no idea when I'm going to eat again so I better store lots of fat. And the next time I do eat because I'm starved I'm going to surely overeat." By skipping meals you also don't get the full 10% benefit of calories burned every time you eat.

Have you ever been on a diet, lost weight, and gained the weight back and then some? If you are a chronic yo-yo dieter (a roller-coaster rider), after many years of highs and lows with your fluctuating weight, your metabolism slows down over time just like the roller-coaster cars do at the end of the ride.

This effect of yo-yo dieting is one of the reasons I encourage you to make a lifestyle change by focusing on eating healthier for the rest of your life rather than going on a roller-coaster, calorie-deprivation diets. The main reason most diets don't work in the long run is because they are not realistic. They are extremely different than what you are accustomed to eating, and they are far too narrow in their choice of foods.

According to Molly Kimball, RD:

> Extra weight causes your body to work harder just to maintain itself at rest, so in most instances the metabolism is always running a bit faster. That's one reason it's always easier to lose weight at the start of a diet and harder later on. When you are very overweight, your metabolism is already running so high any small cut in calories will result in immediate loss. Then you lose significant amounts of body fat and muscle, and your body needs fewer calories to sustain itself. That helps to explain why it's so easy to regain weight after you've worked to lose it (Bounchez, 2006).

Please check with your primary care provider (PCP) if you think you have a slow metabolism because of a possible medical condition such as hypothyroidism.

Finding Fitness

The *International Journal of Obesity* (July 20, 2004), reporting on the Nurses' Health Study noted that mild weight cyclers gained an average of 6.7 pounds and severe weight cyclers gained approximately 10.3 pounds more than non-cyclers. The conclusion was weight cycling was associated with greater weight gain, less physical activity, and a higher prevalence of binge eating. (The Nurses' Health Study [www.channing.harvard.edu/nhs] began in 1976 and has involved more than 200,000 nurses in its research.) Weight cycling is yo-yo dieting where a nurse has lost weight and gained it back and sometimes more over many years of unhealthy dieting. Since this study was performed specifically with nurses I thought it was relevant in showing the negative unhealthy effects of yo-yo dieting over time.

Fast Foods and Slow Foods

Fast Foods = Slow Metabolism

Slow Foods = Fast Metabolism

I characterize *fast foods* as any unhealthy foods that are digested quickly and that rapidly spike your blood sugar and then lower it. Fast foods are unhealthy, calorie-laden, saturated- and trans-fat foods. These types of unhealthy food groups can negatively impact your hormones and cause a sluggish slow unbalanced metabolism. I'm talking caterpillar slow.

Fast foods are processed foods that lack nutritional value, contain an overload of chemical preservatives, and added sugar. These include cakes, cookies, sodas, white breads, potato chips, caffeine, alcohol, and so on. Of course, fast foods can also be found at—you guessed it—fast food restaurants.

I characterize *slow foods* as hormonally balanced, energy-dense fiber foods that your body digests slower. You are fuller longer, and your blood sugar doesn't spike and plummet as it does with fast foods. These foods are more natural and can help speed up your metabolism. They include whole grains, veggies, fruit, beans, fish, lean meats, tofu, and essential fats like avocado, nut, and olive oil.

The good news is that no matter how much you have compromised your metabolism, when you begin creating a healthier lifestyle, you have the capacity to reenergize your metabolism, making it more balanced and functional. One of the great benefits, besides improving your overall health, is how dramatically your energy level improves once you replace fast foods with slow foods.

Exercise: Natural Ways to Boost and Balance Your Metabolism

I feel at my best when:

_____ I eat at least every 3 to 4 hours: three healthy portion–sized meals and at least one healthy snack daily to benefit the 10% thermic effect of food metabolic rate. Thermic effect of food is the energy expenditure above resting metabolic rate due to the processing of food for storage and use. Or, as noted earlier in this chapter, it is the calories expended every time you eat.

_____ I eat natural slow foods that are energy enhanced instead of unhealthy fast foods.

_____ I place aerobic fitness into my schedule such as walking, swimming, biking, and so on. It helps burn calories in the short term and benefits up to 30% of my metabolic rate.

_____ I weight train to build muscle, which burns calories even at rest and benefits up to 30% of my metabolic rate.

_____ I drink plenty of water to help with my digestive system.

_____ I eat breakfast to boost my metabolism when it is the fastest in the morning.

_____ I don't go on a starvation diet under 1,200 calories which signals my body to slow my metabolism and store fat.

_____ I don't skip meals because it slows down my metabolism, lowers my blood sugar, and sets me up to overeat at the next meal.

Your metabolism is your best friend. Treat it well, and it repays you with loyal support of increased energy, better health, and more consistent weight management!

Discharge Care Plan

For fun, to be formally discharged from this chapter, please use your nurse prioritizing skills to reinforce some of the key messages of the chapter. Place what you think would be the correct prioritized number 1-4 in order of importance next to the corresponding letter.

A. __ I schedule in weight training to build muscle and aerobic fitness to help raise my metabolism, and this benefits me up to 30% of my metabolic rate.

B. __ I do not skip meals because it can slow down my metabolism.

C. __ I eat healthy portion–sized meals at least every 3–4 hours and one healthy snack daily to benefit the 10% thermic effect of my food.

D. __ My metabolism is like the Titanic—sinking fast!

Congratulations! You have earned a Golden Nightingale Wellness Wing by completing the interactive portions of the chapter!

(A = 3; B =1; C = 2; D = 4)

5

"If I have the power to nurture patients' health and well-being, then I have the power to nurture my own health and well-being."

–Gary Scholar

In Control:
Managing Blood Pressure, Cholesterol, and Blood Sugar

This chapter is for those with high blood pressure, high cholesterol, and/or diabetes, but it is also for you—whether or not you suffer from those conditions—as support for those in your life who do. It is also a checklist for those nurses who want to prevent inherited high blood pressure, high cholesterol, or high blood sugar or for nurses who already have these health conditions and want to effectively manage them. The treatments in this chapter are compiled from the American Heart Association, American Diabetes Association, WebMD, and the Mayo Clinic.

Maintaining Healthy Blood Pressure

Numbers to watch: You want your blood pressure to be no higher than 120/80.

I feel at my best when I:

___ Schedule a blood pressure screening

___ Consult my primary care provider (PCP) about medications if needed

___ Consult my PCP before starting an exercise program

___ Have my blood pressure checked regularly

LIVEWELL

Body Fat: Loose connective tissue composed of adipocytes

Body Fat Percentage: Percentage of fat your body contains. It is the weight of your fat divided by your total weight.

BMI (Body Mass Index): Estimates ideal weight based on height and weight. (The drawback with BMI is that it doesn't account for how much muscle and fat a person is made up of.)

Consider the following as you strive to maintain healthy blood pressure:

- Losing body fat percentage reduces workload on your heart. Your body fat percentage should be in these healthy ranges:

  - Men 14-17% for fitness, 18-26% for acceptable good health.

  - Women 21 -24% for fitness, 25% - 30% for acceptable good health.

- If you are significantly over the acceptable good health range, then losing 5-10% of your body fat can reduce workload on your heart which would significantly improve your blood pressure.

- Three-quarters (75%) of your salt intake comes from processed foods. Limit processed food intake. Eat whole, natural foods and homemade foods without added salt.

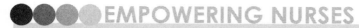

EMPOWERING NURSES

The Salt of the Earth

The real difference between table salt and sea salt is processing, taste, and texture. They are both primarily sodium and chloride. Sea salt is made with less processing and is often touted as a more natural choice. There are other minerals that remain in sea salt that alter its taste and give it a more coarse texture. Some find they don't need as much sea salt as they do with table salt because of the taste. Thus, they use less salt overall. That is a good thing. However, you still need to watch the amount of sea salt you use.

All table salt has been processed extensively and has had iodine added to it. Salt substitutes often include those made of potassium chloride instead of sodium. These are often blends of herbs and spices that leave out salt.

Because our food supply is so salt laden, the recommendation is to use salt alternatives in the form of fresh and dried herbs and spices and less salt when cooking. Avoid salting your food completely at the table.

Consider the following as you strive to maintain healthy blood pressure:

- Decrease sodium to 1,200 mg or less per day. The average intake is more than 3,500 mg per day. Sodium accumulates in blood vessels which can cause higher blood pressure in those who are salt sensitive.

Consider the following as you strive to maintain healthy blood pressure:

- Eat foods high in potassium, calcium, magnesium, and fiber: vegetables, fruits, whole grains, legumes, raw almonds, walnuts, and so on.

LIVEWELL

Ah, Nuts!

Nuts are wonderful in many ways. They provide a lot of healthy fats and fiber along with some protein. However, 1 cup of mixed nuts from a can provide 800 calories and 1,100 mg of sodium. This is similar for peanuts and sunflower seeds. I encourage people to buy raw from the health food store, dry roasted without salt, or unsalted fresh peanuts out of the shell. Eat in 1/4 cup serving amounts as toppings or part of snacks.

LIVEWELL

Roast Your Own

Purchase raw (unseasoned and uncooked) nuts—almonds, walnuts, cashews, pecans, macadamia, Brazil nuts, and so on—and seeds—sunflower and pumpkin—at health food stores and make your own inexpensive, low sodium snacks while spicing them up.

Preheat the oven to between 170-200 degrees. Mix the raw nuts or seeds with your choice of dressing—low sodium soy or tamari sauce, balsamic vinegar, or your favorite low sodium/low fat salad dressing and any non-salt seasoning like herbs—and place them on a large baking sheet. Place the baking sheet in the oven for 20 minutes while turning the nuts or seeds every 5 minutes or so. (Low temperatures should always be used to keep the natural nut and seed oils stable.) You will be amazed at how tasty and inexpensive they are. For the same cost as buying a small can of cocktail or dry roasted nuts at your grocery, you can usually end up with a pound or more of delicious low-sodium, low-fat snacking nuts.

- Avoid foods with high saturated fats, cholesterol, and trans fats that can block arteries.

  - Hot dogs, processed lunch meats, sausage, salami, and dairy products like cheese are high in saturated fats.

  - Cholesterol is found mostly in meat, poultry, and dairy products, including full fat milk, chicken skin, and marbelized meats. Shrimp is somewhat high in cholesterol.

  - Trans fats are found in processed foods such as crackers, candies, cookies, chips, and so on.

- Exercise 30–45 minutes at least 3 times a week. Everyone's heard it a million times by now, but if you can't do anything else, walk!

- Limit alcohol to no more than one drink per day.

  - You may have a tendency to eat more, unconsciously, when drinking. Drinks themselves can have up to 700 calories if they contain sweet mixers (daiquiris, margaritas, and so on.) This high calorie intake can contribute to excess weight gain. Alcohol also inhibits ADH (anti-diuretic hormone), which allows the blood to absorb adequate fluid. So the fluid that should be entering the blood stream becomes part of urine, and frequent urination associated with drinking leaves a person low on overall fluid. So in a world where many of us are already under hydrated, drinking can contribute to further dehydration, headaches, and so on.

LIVEWELL

Livening Up Your H_2O

If you are bored with plain water, give yourself a flavored treat by using lemons or limes. Squeezing or juicing half a lemon or lime in your water will give you a stronger flavor, however just dropping a slice of lemon in your water will give you a subtle citrus flavor. Another good option is to use frozen fruits (peaches, mangoes, and pineapples) and berries (raspberries, blueberries, and strawberries) as ice cubes. Herbal teas can add just a bit of flavor to even cool or iced drinks. Just put a tea bag in your water bottle in the morning. Look for interesting flavor combinations. Good ones are lemon-ginger, peach, mixed berry, and tropical fruit. These add flavor and a hint of sophistication without the cost in calories and dehydration.

- Quit smoking. Smoking can constrict your blood vessels, along with the other well-documented damaging health effects.

- Take blood pressure medication as directed by your PCP.

- Manage your stress with relaxation techniques: deep breathing, meditation, Tai Chi, yoga, prayer, and so on. Do your own research for relaxation techniques that work for you. Measure your pulse rate before and after Yoga, Tai Chi, meditation, or deep breathing to confirm that the relaxation technique is working for you. You can keep a journal of your measurements to watch how it lowers your pulse rate over a long period of time. You can do the same with knitting, gardening, reading, taking a warm soothing bath, and so on. When driving or stuck in traffic instead of listening to the news on the radio, play a favorite music CD and take your pulse before and after. Compare your results to when you're listening to the news.

- Manage your stress by getting your needs met (see Chapter 3 for more on getting your needs met).

- Get a good night's sleep. Insomnia can affect your blood pressure.

- Drink plenty of water to avoid dehydration.

  (Compiled from the Mayo Clinic, 2008, and WebMD, n.d.)

Maintaining Healthy Cholesterol

Numbers to watch:

- Total cholesterol should be less than 200 milligrams per deciliter (mg/dl).

- High-density lipoprotein (HDL) should be above 50 mg/dl for women and above 40 mg/dl for men.

- Low-density lipoprotein (LDL) should be under 130 mg/dl.

- Triglycerides should be under 150 mg/dl.

I feel at my best when I:

__ Schedule a cholesterol screening

__ Consult my PCP for proper treatment if I need medication and before starting an exercise program

As hormones decrease and metabolism slows with age, the body processes cholesterol less efficiently. Consider the following things as you strive to maintain healthy cholesterol:

- Decrease added sugars. Excess insulin can stimulate the liver to produce more LDL cholesterol.

- Avoid meat and dairy products that are high in saturated fat and cholesterol.

- If you choose to eat meat, choose lean cuts and trim off excess fat.

- Exercise at least 30–45 minutes 3 times a week to raise your HDL cholesterol and lower your LDL.

- Consume less than 200 milligrams of cholesterol a day.

- Eat foods high in Omega 3 fats: cold water fish, walnuts, and so on.

●●●●●EMPOWERING NURSES

Okinawa Program

The book *The Okinawa Program* by Bradley Willcox, MD, Craig Willcox, PhD, and Makoto Suzuki, MD, is based on a landmark 25 year study. The researchers compared Okinawan diets with American diets. The Okinawans are one of the longest living people in the world with one of the highest qualities of life and health. According to the book (2002, pg.71), if Americans lived and ate like Okinawans, 80% of our nation's coronary care units and one third of cancer wards would be shut down.

American Diet—% by weight of particular foods
Grains 11%
Omega 3 foods (e.g., fish) 1%
Meat/poultry and eggs 29%
Calcium rich foods (e.g., dairy) 23%
Vegetables 16%
Fruits 20%
Flavonoid rich foods (e.g., soy) 1%

Okinawan Diet
Grains 32%
Omega 3 foods (e.g., fish) 11%
Meat/poultry and eggs 3%
Calcium rich foods (e.g., dairy) 2%
Vegetables 34%
Fruits 6%
Flavonoid rich foods (e.g., soy) 12%

- Avoid foods with trans fats. Trans fats have been found to raise LDL cholesterol levels, raising the risk of heart disease.

- Lose excess body fat percentage.

- Choose high-fiber foods: beans, whole grains, oatmeal, fruits, vegetables, and so on. Consume 20–25 grams of fiber per day. Example of a 25 gram fiber day: 1/2 cup of steel cup oats (8 grams of fiber), 1 ounce fresh almonds (3 grams fiber), 1 banana (3 grams fiber), 1 whole grain tortilla (3 grams fiber), 1/2 cup of black beans (7 grams of fiber), 1 fresh pear (5 grams fiber). Fruits, vegetables, whole grains, and nuts/beans can get you your recommended level of fiber.

LIVEWELL

Omega 3 fatty acids are important to the flexibility of cell walls and hold anti-inflammation properties. They are found in flax, canola oil, and fatty fish. Omega 6 fatty acids are usually abundant in the American diet. They are found in a variety of oils but unfortunately are often hydrogenated and added to many foods. Omega 9 fatty acids are found in olive oil, avocados, nuts, and seeds. Overall health can be improved through adequate Omega 3 and Omega 9 intakes.

- Quit smoking, which helps raise your HDL. Quitting smoking raises your good cholesterol HDL. When you are smoking it lowers your HDL.

- Reduce your stress by getting your needs met and by using relaxation techniques: deep breathing, meditation, Tai Chi, yoga, and so on.

   (Compiled from the American Heart Association, n.d., and WebMD, 2007.)

Maintaining Healthy Blood Sugar

Numbers to watch: Try to maintain a fasting blood sugar under 100 mg/dl.

I feel at my best when I:

__ Schedule a blood sugar screening

__ Consult with my PCP for proper treatment if medication is needed and before I start an exercise program.

To decrease added sugar, consider the following:

- Select natural whole foods; avoid processed foods.

- Eat unsaturated healthy fats—found in cold water fish, flaxseed, and so on—that help stabilize insulin.

- Avoid soft drinks, caffeine, and alcohol.

- Consume 20–25 grams of fiber per day. Fiber raises blood sugar more gradually. It's found in vegetables, most fruits, whole grains, beans, and brown rice.

- Lose body fat if you are overweight.

- Don't skip meals. Blood sugar drops creating a roller coaster effect on your blood sugar level. Often you end up binging on food to spike your blood sugar back up.

LIVEWELL

Fresh or Frozen?

Fresh is always the most nutrient rich. However, frozen forms can be close. Vegetables are blanched immediately before being frozen to kill bacteria growth and slow ripening. A small amount of nutrition is lost during this process but probably no more than fresh loses during shipping and storage. Also, sodium content may be higher in frozen and canned foods. Always read your food label for the sodium content.

- Eat smaller meals throughout the day with healthy snacks in between to keep your blood sugar level. Whenever possible a good combination of complex carbohydrate and proteins seems to keep blood sugars even throughout the day.

  Baked chips and salsa

  Whole wheat crackers and natural peanut or almond butter

  $\frac{1}{2}$ whole wheat pita with 1-2 tablespoons hummus

  Red pepper slices with low fat veggie dip

  Low fat, sugar free yogurt

  Natural peanut or almond butter on whole grain bread

  1 cup cantaloupe and $\frac{1}{4}$ cup low fat cottage cheese

  Sugar free gelatin and fat free whipped topping

- Exercise at least 30–45 minutes every week. This exercise helps insulin work more efficiently. The more muscle you develop, the more sugar you remove from your bloodstream without taxing the pancreas.

- Quit smoking.

Compiled from the American Diabetes Association, n.d., retrieved from http://www.diabetes.org/ diabetes-basics/prevention and http://www.diabetes.org/food-and-fitness/)

Discharge Care Plan

Please use your nursing prioritizing skill to reinforce some of the messages of this chapter. Place what you think are the correct prioritized numbers 1-4 in order of importance next to the corresponding letter.

A. __ Numbers to watch: B.P. 120/80; blood sugar under 100 mg/dl; total cholesterol under 200 mg/dl; HDL above 50 mg/dl for women and above 40 mg/dl for men; LDL under 130 mg/dl; and triglycerides under 150 mg/dl

B. __ Exercise 30–45 minutes at least 3 times a week to help manage your blood sugar, blood pressure, and cholesterol

C. __ Select whole, natural foods. Avoid highly processed foods, added sugars, high saturated fats, and trans fats, and reduce sodium intake.

D. __ Numbers to watch: 6, 10, 12, 22, 26, 50. Winning lotto numbers!

Congratulations! You have earned a Golden Nightingale Wellness Wing by completing the interactive portions of the chapter.

(A = 1; B = 3; C = 2; D = 4)

6

"Since I made exercise a regular part of my life, my energy level and my feeling of well-being are off the charts! Schedule it, love it, do it. You deserve it!"

–Gary Scholar

How ER (Exercising Regularly) Can Help Keep You Out of the ED (Emergency Department)

Adding a regular fitness routine into an already hectic schedule can be difficult. I hear this over and over again from nurses. You can compare it to trying to cram your feet into shoes that are two sizes too small—no matter how much you may want to fit into those shoes, there's simply no room!

It's always a good idea to consult your primary care provider before starting a new exercise program, including the one in this chapter. If you experience discomfort during exercise, you should discontinue what you are doing and consult your care provider.

The ultimate cure for lack of motivation is to provide you with inspiring and empowering reasons to make fitness a regular part of your lifestyle.

Here are examples of reasons from one nurse: I will schedule in fitness I enjoy because

1. Fitness is something special to do just for myself which breaks the unhealthy cycle of being a Type E nurse personality.

2. Fitness gives me a sense of control over my health, weight, and well-being.

3. Fitness helps me manage my stress levels by engaging my mind and lowering my stress hormones of cortisol and stimulating the production of endorphins that will produce feelings of well-being.

4. Fitness gives me a sense of achievement when a goal is reached.

5. Fitness heightens my sense of self-esteem by allowing me to feel better about my body image.

6. Fitness increases my energy level, raises my metabolism, induces quality of sleep, and sharpens my mental focus.

Results is the ultimate cure for the lack of finding time to schedule exercise. If you make the commitment, I promise that you will begin to feel the sense of empowerment inherent in the activity and the routine of exercising after only 2 weeks. You deserve it!

If you are one of the nurses who believe you don't have time to exercise, think about the fact that not exercising increases your "time" of feeling overwhelmed, stressed out, and exhausted.

This is true because for every minute you exercise you decrease your stress hormone of cortisol secretion, reduce muscle tension, and raise your metabolism which helps increase your energy level. You also increase production of your feel good neurotransmitters of endorphins. By nurturing yourself with exercise, you help manage your feeling of not being in control of certain areas of your life.

LIVEWELL

"I have two boys, one of whom isn't in school yet. I take care of the family all day and then work the night shift. Needless to say, I am completely exhausted most of the time. I know if I exercised, I would have more energy. But I can't even get myself started at that point."

–Melissa, Hospital RN

"As a nurse, I want to take care of everybody; that is my nature. Everyone and everything has to be taken care of before I think about myself. By the time I get around to 'my time' I'm too tired, and I just want to get home, take a shower, and sit. I sure don't feel like exercising. A walk? Please! I've been running around at work all day!"

–Carmen, Clinical and Hospital RN

"When it comes to exercise, I'm too tired before work. I wake up, crawl to the bathroom, get ready, and then race off to work. During work, I don't even have time to pee. After work, I'm so pooped I don't have the energy to even walk my dog."

–Hope, ED nurse, single with no children

Do What You Love, and Fitness Will Come

When you make defeating comments, you are essentially saying to yourself that you are not important enough to invest time in and don't deserve to feel better. I firmly believe you deserve to feel better. This is your time to take charge and use your assertiveness to find the healthy and happy you that's hiding inside. Become your own best patient. Are you one of the nurses who believe you get all the exercise you need walking while on duty at the hospital? Not so fast! The walking you do on your shifts at work and the fitness necessary to raise your energy level are vastly different. The walking you do on your shift is a low level of intensity that does not raise your heart rate for a sustained period of time as it would in aerobic exercise. It also does not significantly raise your metabolism and endorphin levels to give your increased energy and feelings of well-being. What walking on your shift does is keep you on your feet all day. Coupled with the stress of the job, the result is exhaustion. Walking your shifts drain you emotionally and physically, but fitness empowers and energizes you.

Two important strategies can help you successfully inject fitness into your life and create a healthier lifestyle:

- Engage in physical activity you enjoy.

- Place your activity into a schedule that works for you.

Assertively engaging in physical activity you enjoy is vital. Otherwise, you can sabotage your own efforts because you won't enjoy the fitness enough to stick with it. In my experience, about half of those who start exercising drop out after 6 months because they don't enjoy it. That percentage is much higher, in my experience, with nurses because of the hectic schedules.

I will use myself as an example. Many years ago some of my friends were competing in 5k, 10k, triathlons, and marathon races. So they encouraged me to race with them. I never enjoyed the workouts, so I would find every excuse under the sun not to train and come race day the only moment I enjoyed was getting a massage afterward! So I learned to just stick to what I enjoy most, which is playing sports. For example, it doesn't matter how busy or tired I am if I'm scheduled to play tennis I can't wait to play. I love it!

LIVEWELL

"I went on vacation and rode a bicycle for the first time in 40 years. When I got back home, I borrowed my daughter-in-law's bike and started riding the streets. I rode 4 days a week, 10–12 miles a day."

–Karen, nurse executive

Working out in a gym might not be your cup of tea. That's why I want you to first find a physical activity that fits your enjoyment level. It could be swimming, dancing, ice skating, tennis, volleyball, golf, biking, yoga, or horseback riding. Whatever activity you love, you should do; you should look forward to both the activity and the time spent doing it.

Take the time to create a list of physical activities you enjoy and research where you can participate in them in an area that's convenient for you.

Activity	Location

The second component to making room for fitness involves placing activity in a schedule that works for you. Remember that any exercise is better than no exercise, but the more you enjoy your workout, the more you will work out; the more you work out, the fitter and healthier you will become.

EMPOWERING NURSES

"I walk approximately three to five times a week with my dog. I also go to a women's gym three times a week. I find this activity makes me feel better, more energized, and I have more restful sleep."

–Andrea, hospital nurse

"I always remind myself that exercise is an important stress reliever. I feel better when I take care of myself. I am happier and have more energy. I work out on my days off, as well as before work. It's early, but I feel so much better at work. And it allows me to spend more time with my family after work. I do 30–45 minutes of cardio—treadmill, elliptical, bike, stair climber—and 30 minutes of weights."

–Sue, hospital nurse

"As a new mom I have purchased a jogging stroller which I hope will motivate me to start jogging. I always find jogging to be invigorating and hope it will help with my energy level with the new baby."

–Jennifer, hospital nurse

"I take short naps on my days off to reenergize myself for my gym workouts."

–Jessica, hospital nurse

●●●●● EMPOWERING NURSES

"I personally always try to go to the gym on my way home from work. This just happens to be the best time for me because my husband is at work, so it doesn't take away from our time together in the evenings. After working out I feel much better about myself and find that I sleep better during the day!"

–Jennifer, night-shift nurse

"On the night I work, I do stretching exercises and jumping jacks. Then I do 25 minutes on the weight machines. In the morning after I work, I go for a 5-mile run 3 times a week. I work out a total of 4–5 times a week."

–Cassandra, hospital nurse

"My shift is from 1 p.m. to 1 a.m. The key for me regarding exercise is consistency. I started working out 10 years ago when I was overweight and pre-diabetic. Now I'm off diabetic meds. I work out for 1 hour 3 times a week or 30 minutes 4 or 5 times a week. I walk on the bike path or use a treadmill."

–Renee, resource nurse

"I worked 3–4 12-hour shifts in the ER. On my days off I worked out. It felt so good I started working out before I went to work. Now I'm working in radiology 5 days a week for 8 hours a day. My workouts consist of 30–45 minutes on the treadmill, bike, elliptical, or stair climber, and 30 minutes of weight training alternating days between upper body and lower body workouts."

–Allison, radiology clinical nurse manager

There are four key components in your ability to schedule fitness into your hectic schedule. The first component is to sit down with your work/life schedule and make a choice that bests fits your personal needs based upon the time of day. Your choices are to schedule fitness in before work, during work, after work, or on a day off. It really all depends on which time gives you the best opportunity to sustain your commitment to regularly exercise. For some nurses that depends on their energy level and convenience of location at that time of day or night.

The second component is creating space in your schedule to accommodate your fitness. That may mean switching a responsibility or activity to another time—or getting rid of something in your schedule that is draining you.

The third component is becoming assertive by setting a healthy boundary in order to consistently keep to your commitment to exercise. That may mean leaving work on time, asking your spouse to make dinner or pick up the kids or you decline an invitation to participate in a community volunteer opportunity.

The fourth component is deciding what type of exercise would be best in your time slot. For example, if you're working nights you may want something (yoga, Pilates, or Tai Chi) that isn't high impact intensity and helps you sleep better.

The fifth component is to give yourself an accountability timeline so you don't sabotage your efforts as to when you will start your fitness plan. You should start your fitness plan within two weeks of finding an activity you will enjoy and the location of where you will engage in the activity.

Benefits of E.R. (Exercising Regularly)

E.R. offers many life benefits, including the following:

- E.R. is a good predictor of long-term weight management because it raises your metabolism.

- The number one reason nurses exercise is for stress relief. E.R. raises your endorphin levels, which calms your mind to better cope with stress and feelings of being overwhelmed. It also creates a huge ripple effect on your family. First, you're a happier person to be around because exercise has a positive effect on your mood. Second, you are modeling for your children that self care is high on your priority list.

- Many nurses report that they feel more energized when they have regular exercise and are more present and focused both in their jobs and in their home life.

- Nurses' self-confidence about their body image also improves with regular exercise.

- One pound of muscle takes up approximately fives times less area then one pound of fat. That's why your clothes fit better when you add muscle through E.R.

- Because of the increased amount of oxygen to the brain, E.R. increases alertness for nurses.

- E.R. eases muscle tension brought on by long, demanding hours at work.

- E.R. helps manage blood pressure, cholesterol, and blood sugar levels.

- E.R. helps promote proper sleep, especially for those nurses working rotating or night shifts.

> The Nurse Health Study reports that no matter how much you weigh, you can reduce your risk of diabetes by being physically active. If you are overweight and have a greater risk of diabetes, you can benefit most from activity. Also, those nurses who walked at least 4 hours a week of sustained exercise had 40% reduction in hip fractures. (Sustained exercise is 30 minutes or more.)

Target Heart Rate

To get your maximum benefit during your aerobic workout (walking, biking, jogging, etc.), you need to train within your target heart rate. You can also choose to take your own pulse while exercising, using the carotid artery on the side of your neck, or you can use a heart rate monitor either on a treadmill, elliptical machine, or you can buy one to place on your arm. Your level of fitness determines where your target heart rate zone is.

Table 6.1   Target heart rate zone.

Beginner or low-fitness level: 50%–60%

Moderate-fitness level: 60%–70%

Advanced-fitness level: 75%–85%

To calculate your target heart rate, for example, if you are a beginner or at a low-fitness level, subtract your age from 220 and multiply this number by .50 and then .60 to find your target heart rate range (or zone) of beats per minute. Your goal is to exercise within your zone or adjust your workout until you get into your zone.

Table 6.2	Formula for determining your target heart rate zone.

220 – age times .50 = lower intensity zone

220 – age times .60 = higher intensity zone

If you are beginning an exercise program, you should be able to talk during your workout without much effort. You can buy a heart rate monitor online or at many sport and retail stores. A great benefit about being a nurse is you already know how to check your own heart rate!

Refuel after working out to keep your blood sugar level. It's best to combine a protein with a complex carbohydrate, for example, an apple with almond butter.

Diabetes and Physical Activity

If you have diabetes and are planning on exercising, please follow the advice given by the American Diabetes Association (www.diabetes.org):

1. Talk to your health care team about which activities are safe for you.

2. Checking your blood glucose before and after you exercise can show you the benefits of the activity, but you can also use the results to prevent low or high blood glucose.

3. If your blood glucose is high before you exercise (above 300), physical activity can make it higher. For those with Type 1 diabetes, if your fasting glucose level is above 250 and you have ketones in your urine, it's best to avoid exercise.

4. Be aware that low blood glucose can occur during or long after physical activity. It occurs most often if you:

   - Take insulin or diabetes medication

   - Skip a meal

   - Exercise a long time

   - Exercise strenuously

5. If low blood glucose is interfering with your exercise routine, eating a snack before you exercise or adjusting your medication can help. Talk to your health care team about what is right for you. During activity, check your blood glucose if you notice symptoms such as hunger, nervousness, shakiness, or sweating.

6. If your blood glucose is low have a half a cup (4 ounces) of fruit juice. After 15 minutes check your blood glucose again. Have another serving of fruit juice and repeat the step until your blood glucose is at least 70.

7. Drink plenty of water before, during, and after activity.

8. Wear a medical ID to protect yourself in case of an emergency.

9. Monitor your feet and toes for sore spots or blisters.

Depression and exercise—Christine Northrup, MD, author of *The Wisdom of Menopause* (2006, pp. 308 -309) writes, "Exercise changes brain chemistry by increasing beta-endorphins, lowering catecholamines, and increasing monoamines, and both aerobic and non-aerobic forms have been shown to be helpful in individuals with mild to moderate depression.

Care Plans

Care plans are a proactive guide for you to follow based on your fitness interest, fitness level, and goals. Care plans should be used for a 3 month duration since that is how long it takes to see significant change and benefits. At the end of the 3 months you will be at a different fitness level and may choose to revise your plan to reflect your new level or so you do not plateau. Incorporating cardio, strength, and flexibility in your care plan will give you the optimal benefits for your health, body, and well-being.

You can integrate the following fitness choices into your fitness care plan:

1. **Low impact:** Tai Chi, yoga, Pilates, and so on

2. **Gym workout:** Cardio: elliptical, treadmill, bike, and so on; strength training: free weights, machines, stability ball, and so on; fitness classes

3. **Cardio:** Walking, jogging, swimming, biking, and so on

4. **Just for fun:** Dance, tennis, volleyball, golf, ice skating, and so on

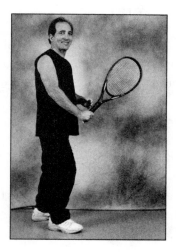

Figure 6.1

Find a fitness activity that you love and do it!

Fit Nurse Care Plan 1

Fit Nurse Care Plan 1 is for a nurse who might or might not have exercised in the past, but has not worked out in the past 3–6 months and needs to start slow by walking. Make sure to get the go ahead to exercise after consulting with your primary care provider.

As a way to calculate your progress rate, you can use a perceived overall energy level of 1–10, 1 being low and 10 being a high energy level.

- Before I begin my Fit Nurse Care Plan 1 my overall energy level is_____.
- My overall energy level after week 5 is _____.
- My overall energy level after week 12 is _____.

Wearing the correct shoes depending on what specific workout or sport you are doing is the single most important equipment choice you can make. If your feet hurt, odds are high that you will be discouraged quickly. The right shoe helps you improve your fitness and decreases the chance of injury. For example, walking shoes should fit securely around your heel and allow your toes to spread when you are pushing off the ground by having a 1/2-thumb distance from your big toe to the tip of your shoe.

Walking

Walk with your chin up and your shoulders held slightly back. Walk so the heel of your foot touches the ground first. Roll your weight forward and push off your big toe. Pump your arms forward as you walk to gain efficient momentum.

Figure 6.2

Proper walking mechanics.

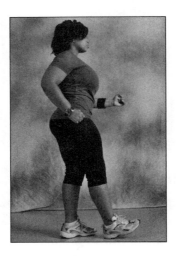

To avoid sore muscles and joints, you should start walking gradually, and don't overdo it. It's a good idea to buy a pedometer to keep track of how far you have walked. If you are walking on a treadmill, start slowly at 2.0 miles per hour and then you can increase it to 3.0 miles per hour. Eventually, if you feel confident, increase to 3.5 miles per hour. Remember these are only guidelines. You should go at your own pace, something you feel comfortable with.

Table 6.3   Walking: 3 to 5 times a week

| | Warm Up | | Cool Down | |
	Walk Slowly	Walk Briskly	Walk Slowly	Total Time
Week 1–2	5 min.	5 min.	5 min.	15 minutes
Week 3–5	5 min.	15 min.	5 min.	25 minutes
Week 6–8	5 min.	25 min.	5 min.	35 minutes
Week 9–12	5 min.	30 min.	5 min.	40 minutes

Every mile you walk is approximately 2,000 steps. Walk with a pedometer to count your steps. The goal for weight management is 10,000 steps or more a day, which equals approximately 4.0 miles.

Inject interval training if you plateau in your workout or for weight management. Change the intensity level, intervals of rest, or type of physical activity. For example, walk moderately for 2 minutes, then walk faster for 3 minutes, and then go back to walking moderately for 2 minutes. This type of interval training burns calories without fatiguing you with constant high-level intensity. One innovative way to add interest to your walking routine is ChiWalking, which blends mind and body into your walking routine (see www.chiwalking.com).

Flexibility

Effective stretching and flexibility exercises help reduce injuries and create a full range of motion without pain and discomfort to your muscles and joints.

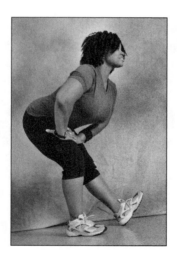

Figure 6.3

Proper flexibility stretching techniques.

Standing with your right heel forward, place your hands on your left knee. Hold for 6–8 seconds so that you feel a slight stretch in the back of your right leg. Repeat on the left leg.

Stand facing a wall about 2 feet or less from it, place your hands chest high on the wall with your right leg bent at a 45-degree angle and your left leg straight. Hold for 6–8 seconds to feel a slight stretch down your left leg. Repeat on the right leg.

Strength Training: Alternate Days—3 days a week.

If you want to, you can add strength training in week 6.

Week 1–8

Without the use of a personal trainer or joining a gym, you can do the following strength exercises anytime and anywhere that provides an opportunity—during your breaks, before or after work, etc.

1. **Chair squats:** Start sitting in an upright chair. Using only the muscles in your legs, proceed to slowly stand and then slowly sit. Repeat 8–10 times.

2. **Wall push-ups:** Stand facing the wall about 2 to 3 feet away, lean forward, placing your hands against the wall chest high and slightly wider than your shoulders. Slowly lower your nose toward the wall and then push away, extending your arms completely. Repeat 8–10 times.

3. **Abdominal crunches:** Lie on your back, hands behind your head for support, knees bent, feet on the floor. Using the muscles in your abdominals, lift your shoulders slowly off the ground while exhaling, and slowly lower down while inhaling. Do not let your head touch the ground until you are done. Repeat 8–10 times.

Week 9–12

For a more comprehensive approach to weight training, there are any number of reputable videos available. I particularly recommend *Shaping up with Weights for Dummies*, or suggest you seek the assistance of a personal trainer if you have never lifted weights before.

An inexpensive approach to strength training and one you could do at home or if you are traveling would be to purchase resistance bands or tubes and an exercise ball. They can be purchased at most general retail and sports store.

There are hundreds of different strength training exercises you can perform with them.

Resistance bands and tubes are made of material that stretches. The further the band or tube stretches, more resistance provided. They come in a variety of resistance from ultra light to maximum strength. They can be used like free weights in that you perform a number of repetitions with them to build up strength, muscular endurance, and help tone your body.

Exercise balls, also called Swiss balls—so named for a group of Swiss physical therapists who used the balls when working with children with cerebral palsy—are very effective. The balls come in a variety of sizes appropriate to a person's size. The instability of the ball challenges your body to improve core muscle strength, range of motion, enhanced balance, and greater flexibility. For example, performing an abdominal crunch with an exercise ball will target your abdominal and back muscles while focusing on maintaining your balance. Another example, I have typed this entire book while sitting on my exercise ball. By doing so it has strengthened my core muscles. Core muscles are located deep in your pelvis, abdomen, trunk, and back.

For women, I also recommend Curves. It is a women-only circuit training gym that has 10,000 locations worldwide. It is not expensive and offers all components for a well-rounded 30 minute workout, which fits perfectly into the hectic schedule of a nurse. It includes both cardio and strength training. It's perfect for the Fit Nurse Care Plan 1 or Fit Nurse Care Plan 2.

Just for Fun

Starting week 1 is the time to do something for the pure fun of it. It can be biking, dancing, or taking your dog for a walk. It can involve your family or friends or just be time for you. For weeks 1–12, allow yourself to integrate at least 1 day a week for something active that's really fun!

Empowered Fitness

Incorporate empowered fitness every once in a while or place it in your weekly schedule. An example of empowered fitness is something I did in the process of writing this book. I took daily walks along Lake Michigan. Walking along the lake shore and looking out onto the breathtaking views of the water empowered my writing and helped my creative process by giving me clarity, and looking out to the vast horizon made me realize the endless possibilities involved in making a difference in the quality of life for nurses. Other examples might be a nature walk, snorkeling, cross country skiing, and so on.

Fit Nurse Care Plan 2

Fit Nurse Care Plan 2 is for the nurse who has been exercising consistently for at least 6 months and is physically ready for more variety and an advanced level of fitness.

As with before, calculate your progress rate using your perceived overall energy level of 1–10, 1 being low and 10 being a high energy level.

- Before I begin my Fit Nurse Care Plan 2 my overall energy level is _____.

- At the end of week 5 my overall energy level is _____.

- At the end of week 12 my overall energy level is _____.

Cardio Fitness

These are activities that get you to your target heart rate while working up a sweat. You should be performing them 3 to 5 times a week.

Week 1–5: Choose your activity of choice, for example, cycling, swimming, boxing, walking, jogging, spin classes, and so on. Set your duration at 40–60 minutes, depending on your level of fitness.

Week 6–12: Choose a new activity so you cross-train your body and you don't get bored.

Flexibility

You should incorporate Tai Chi, yoga, or Pilates at least once into your weekly schedule in place of a cardio activity. They are the optimal balance of total stretching and relaxation.

Strength Training

Fit Nurse Care Plan 2 assumes you are familiar with weight training.

Week 1–8

Weight train two or three times a week. Make sure you skip at least a day in between to give your muscles a chance to recover. It is your choice if you want to work alternate days on your upper and lower body because of time constraints or if you want to perform it on the same day.

Performing a total body strength training workout may be good if you are just beginning because it gets your body use to different exercises. But you may notice over time you have reached a plateau as far as your level of workout. The advantage of performing a lower and upper body training session on different days is that it will give you the time and energy to focus on specific muscle groups and add a number of reps or weight.

Perform 8–12 repetitions, 1–2 sets of each exercise. The weight should be challenging enough that it gets tough around the 10th repetition, but not too challenging that you cannot complete the set. Please perform your sets slowly with proper mechanics that help increase your conditioning and prevent injury. So many times individuals perform their weight training too quickly.

Strength training tips to avoid injury:

1. Always warm up your muscles first by performing 10-15 minutes of cardio exercise on a treadmill, elliptical machine, or walking in place.

2. Use a spotter when lifting a heavy weight.

3. Do not lift more weight than you can handle as far as amount of weight or number of reps.

4. Allow 2-3 minutes between sets to rest your muscles.

5. Perform your weight training exercise slowly through the full range of motion. This will make your muscles work harder while at the same time avoiding injury.

Use the following instructions to lift weights for the major muscle groups:

1. **Bicep curls:** Elbows to side, curl your arms up, exhaling on the way up.

2. **Triceps extensions:** Lift your elbow to the back; extend your arm fully.

3. **Chest press:** Lying on your back, extend your arms chest high.

4. **Seated row for your back:** Sitting, pull your arms in, close to your body.

5. **Leg extensions for the quadriceps:** Sitting, extend your legs fully.

6. **Leg curls for the hamstrings:** Sitting, curl your legs to your glutes.

7. **Side-lying adduction (inner thighs):** Lie on your left side, cross your right leg over your extended left leg, and place your right foot in front of your left knee. Slowly lift your left leg up and then slowly down. Repeat 8–10 times and turn over and repeat on the other side.

8. **Side-lying abduction (outer thighs):** Lie on your left side, bend your left leg under your right leg, lift straight up and then slowly down. Repeat 8–10 times and turn over and repeat on the other side.

For more toned upper arms, try the following:

1. **Triceps push-downs** (for use with weight systems at gym): Face a high pulley on a weight machine with your feet shoulder width apart and start with the bar chin high and your upper arms angled slightly. Bring your elbows down in alignment with your body, slowly pushing the bar down. Then slowly let the bar up to the beginning position.

2 **Dumbbell hammer curl:** Put two dumbbells to your side, palms facing in, arms straight, elbows to your side. Raise one dumbbell until your forearm is vertical and your thumb faces your shoulder. Lower to the starting position and repeat using your other arm.

Weeks 9–12

Either increase your resistance by adding a little more weight to each exercise or increase the number of reps or sets you perform. You can also get in the habit of performing abdominal crunches daily to help strengthen your core muscles.

Just for Fun

Integrate a fun activity—dance, tennis, volleyball, ice skating, and so on—into your weekly schedule. It can take the place of your cardio fitness workouts. .

For those nurses who are in good shape, to stay motivated give yourself a big goal to walk or run a 5 or 10k race, marathon, triathlon, or a Breast Cancer walk or run.

DVDs are a wonderful way to workout at home or when you travel. There are hundreds of fitness Web sites online that sell fitness DVDs. You can choose fitness DVDs based on your interest and goal. For example, if you are a night shift nurse and interested in doing yoga before your shift and right after your shift, you may want to check out the Gaiam Web site (www.gaiam.com) which has DVDs for AM/PM yoga. If you need a Web site that has many fitness DVDs to choose from you can check out www.CollageVideo.com. Consider an online search for DVD reviews. It can be helpful to see what others are saying about particular videos.

Scheduling

Your long demanding hours can make it difficult to include fitness into your weekly schedule. Here are examples of how you can be assertive in placing regular exercise into your nursing lifestyle.

12-Hour Shift

If you are working three 12-hour shifts with the rest of the days off, you might want to consider these fitness options:

1. Option 1: Exercise only on your days off. You can schedule in three fun workouts that you enjoy. Determine what time of day works best for you.

2. Option 2: To give you more energy during your shift, schedule your workout before your shift starts, even if it means getting up earlier.

3. Option 3: To give you more energy for your days off, schedule your workout after you are done working.

If you are doing option two or three, you might find it easier because of your energy level to schedule in low impact fitness like Tai Chi, yoga, or Pilates.

Night Shift

Night shift is the most difficult shift to chart for fitness because of the unnatural sleep patterns and exhaustion. So I'm going to leave this to the experts—the actual nurses who are currently working out during the night shift.

1. **Option 1:** Many nurses have reported working out after they are done with their shift and before they go home. They explain it helps with their energy level when they do get home and also helps with more restful sleep. They are also working out on their days off.

2. **Option 2:** Work out with low impact after work (Tai Chi, yoga, and Pilates) so it is easier to get to sleep. Save your higher impact workouts for your days off.

3. **Option 3:** Twenty minutes of aerobic exercise before you start your shift can give you more energy during your shift.

Exercise breaks during work can help maintain alertness.

Traveling Nurse

If you are a nurse traveling to different cities, you might want to consider these fitness options:

1. **Option 1:** Watch FitTV, a TV channel that focuses on fitness and offers many fitness programs for all fitness levels. Bring along resistance bands (Thera Bands) or fitness tubes that are lightweight and can travel with you wherever you go, fitting in your suitcase. They are for strength training exercises. They can be purchased at many sports and general retail stores at reasonable prices. You can also travel with a portable DVD player to exercise with your favorite fitness DVD.

2. **Option 2:** Buy a membership at national fitness facilities like Curves or World Gym so you have a place to work out no matter where you travel.

3. **Option 3:** Walk and see the sights at your new location.

Routines for E.R.

The following sections constitute a quick snapshot of different routines for E.R. you might want to schedule into creating a healthier lifestyle. Pick one or do them all. For a complete exercise routine, work with a personal trainer, sign up with a fitness class, or buy a workout DVD.

Please talk to your primary care provider (PCP) before trying any of the following exercise routines to see if they are right for you. Many times beginners to a new exercise overdo it. Be cautious if you have never had prior experience in regular exercise. Take it slow and easy. If something bothers you, please stop the exercising immediately. The goal is to shift your lifestyle, and any injury, no matter how small, can derail you from that goal.

Tai Chi

Tai Chi classes exist in a long form or short form. However, because of nurses' hectic schedules, schedules that create a lack of time and energy, I've created Gary's form of Tai Chi specifically for nurses. You can perform my Tai Chi anywhere, even in the middle of your shift, at your clinic, or if you're a school nurse in your office. It just takes a few minutes, it's easy, and the great benefit for a nurse is that it's not taxing but gently energizing.

Tai Chi is an ancient Chinese movement-based meditation that is wonderful for nurses because any nurse can do it, no matter age, weight, fitness, or specific health issues. It is wonderful for nurses who are experiencing arthritis. Tai Chi comprises slow flowing movements that quiet your mind and improve your strength, flexibility, balance, and coordination. For a nurse, it helps manage your stress by helping you learn to relax and breathe more deeply. It also makes you connect to your body in a mindful way. If you can, choose soothing music to play along as you perform your routine.

To make sure you are properly breathing from your diaphragm, place your right hand on your abdomen and your left hand on your chest. Breathe into your abdomen to draw your belly up. As you feel your right hand rise up in the air, your left hand on your chest should rise minimally. Exhale and feel your abdomen recede.

Every gentle movement is performed three times in a row.

Figure 6.4

Beginning pose for Tai Chi.

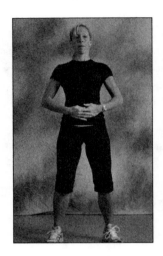

1. **Beginning pose:** Place your hands, cupped over each other, lightly on your belly. Place your feet shoulder-width apart. Take three deep breathes from your dia-phragm. Relax your body by breathing in good thoughts and breathing out all the feel-ings of stress and being over-whelmed. Move smoothly through your slow fluid movements.

Figure 6.5

Tracing fitness Tai Chi movement.

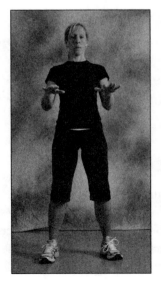

2. **Tracing fitness:** Bring your arms to your side and gently raise them up palms down chest high and bend them at the elbows and slowly press down. Repeat three times.

Figure 6.6

Tracing food plate Tai Chi movement.

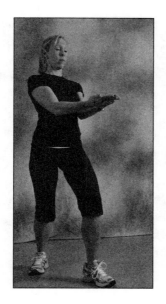

3. **Tracing food plate:** Place one foot in front of the other at a 45 degree angle. Your front knee is slightly bent, the knee is over the ankle, and your front foot should bear more weight than the back foot. Your arms are chest high. With your palms up and hands slightly touching one another, pretend you are tracing a round plate of delicious, healthy food. Repeat three times. Now gently place your other foot in front at a 45 degree angle and repeat tracing your plate three times.

Figure 6.7

Tracing self care circle Tai Chi movement.

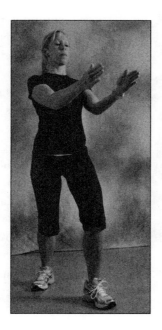

4. **Tracing self care circle:** Pretend you are tracing a large vertical circle (like a big marching drum) with both hands and arms parallel. This signifies your commitment to your own self care. Repeat three times. Now gently place your other foot at a 45 degree angle and repeat tracing self care circle three times.

Figure 6.8

Tracing
healthy
boundary
setting
Tai Chi
movement.

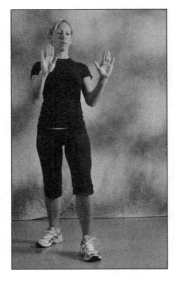

5. **Tracing healthy boundary setting:** Bend your arms chest high. Your hands are upright in the push position, and push away from you and then bring your hands back toward you. Repeat three times. Now gently place your other foot at a 45 degree angle and repeat, tracing your healthy boundary setting three times.

Figure 6.9

Tracing
weight
off your
shoulders
Tai Chi
movement.

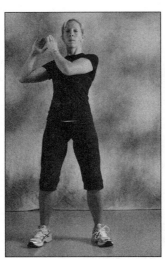

6. **Tracing weight off your shoulders:** Gently change your feet position to shoulder-width apart. Place your open hands above your shoulders. Pretend your hands are holding a huge weight on your shoulders. It signifies taking the weight of responsibility off your shoulders. Now gently take the weight off your shoulders and move it in a large circle with both hands. Repeat three times. Then position the weight on your other shoulder and repeat three times.

Figure 6.10

Return to beginning pose.

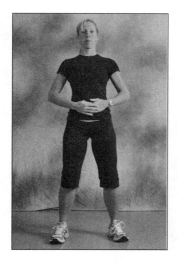

7. Beginning pose: Gently move your hands to your belly, go back to your beginning pose, and breathe deeply three times.

Ahhh . . . don't you feel better now?

Yoga/Pilates

Yoga/Pilates are mind/body exercises that make you feel more relaxed and centered. They create strong, lean, sculpted muscles that also help strengthen your core muscles, which are very important for a nurse. A strong core helps strengthen your back and prevent the chronic back pain so many nurses experience.

1. **Downward Dog:** Begin on your hands and knees, shoulders directly over wrists, hips directly over your knees. Inhale. On the exhale, curl your toes under, lifting your tailbone up toward the sky, pressing your chest and head through your arms. Hold the position and continue to breathe. Hold for 1–3 minutes, breathing deeply from your diaphragm as you hold the pose.

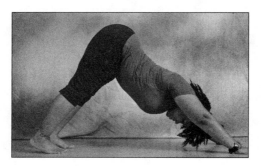

Figure 6.11

Downward dog pose.

2. **Warrior II:** Stand with your right arm forward, left arm backward, and your weight evenly distributed between each leg. Inhale, exhale, and bend your front knee (right knee), keeping your back leg straight and your toes angled slightly inward. Hold for 1–3 minutes, breathing deeply from your diaphragm as you hold the pose.

Figure 6.12

Warrior II
pose.

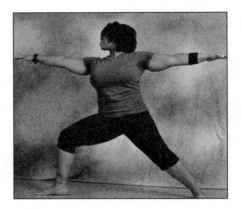

3. **Triangle:** Begin the same as you did for Warrior II. Inhale. While exhaling, slowly lower your right arm down toward your inner right leg, either placing your hand on the floor or your leg. Hold for 1–3 minutes, breathing deeply from your diaphragm as you hold the pose.

Figure 6.13

Triangle
pose.

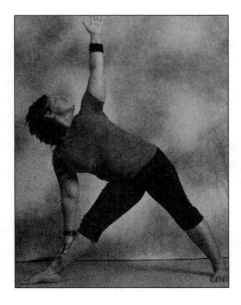

4. **Extended Angle:** Begin the same as you did for Warrior II and Triangle. Inhale. While exhaling, bend your front knee (right knee), place your front elbow gently on your front thigh, and reach opposite arm overhead. Hold for 1–3 minutes, breathing deeply from your diaphragm as you hold the pose.

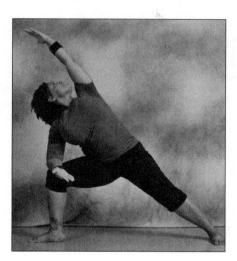

Figure 6.14

Extended angle pose.

5. **Table Top:** Sit with your hands placed slightly behind the hips, fingertips pointing toward your body. Inhale your breath, and while exhaling, lift your hips and buttocks off the ground, looking up toward the sky. Continue to breathe while holding the pose.

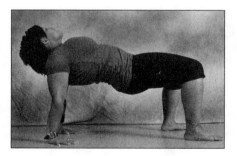

Figure 6.15

Table top pose.

6. **Twists:** Sitting, cross one leg over the other, inhale, exhale, and slowly twist your body toward the crossed over leg.

Figure 6.16

Twist pose.

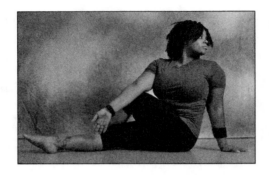

I recommend the books *Yoga for Nurses*, by Ingrid Kollak, a yoga expert and a registered nurse, and Brooke Silver's *Pilates Weight Loss for Beginners*.

Boxing Techniques

For fun, I thought I'd give you a great one-two punch aerobic exercise to relieve some of your nursing stress.

1. **Jab:** Begin in the ready stance, feet hip-width apart, elbows close to ribs, fists protecting your face. Lead with your knuckles, extend your arm forward from the elbow. Follow through with your shoulder and hip.

Figures 6.17-6.19

Jab.

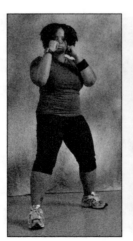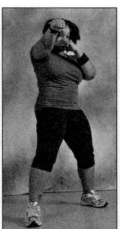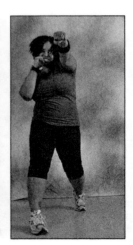

Figures 6.20

Uppercut.

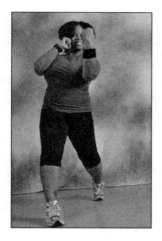

2. **Uppercut:** Begin in the ready stance, arms close to your body. Lead with your knuckles, extend your arm in an upward motion in front of the body. End at the chin level. Follow through with your shoulder and hip.

Figures 6.21

Hook.

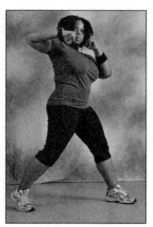

3. **Hook:** Begin in the ready stance, arms close to your body. Lift your elbow as your fist rotates across the front of your body with a gliding motion. Follow through with your shoulder, hip, and knee. End at the opposite shoulder.

Figures 6.22

Elbow strike.

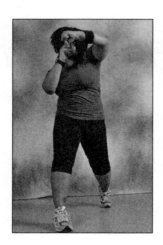

4. **Elbow Strike:** Begin in the ready stance, arms close to your body. Lift your elbow, keeping your fists close together, and thrust your elbow to the side in strike motion. Return to the ready stance.

Strength Training

I'm getting you ready for the upcoming Nurse Olympics. Strength training has the ability to reshape your body and help you lose weight. The following strength training exercises comprise three exercises for the upper body and three for the lower body. Move slowly and deliberately through each exercise so your muscle gets the most benefit from each move and so you don't injure yourself.

Figures 6.23

Bicep curl.

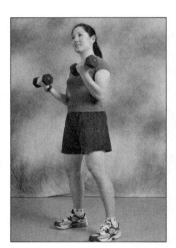

1. **Bicep curl:** Stand with your arms down by your sides. Exhale while curling the weights up toward your shoulders. Lower your arms while inhaling and repeat.

Figures 6.24

Triceps kickback.

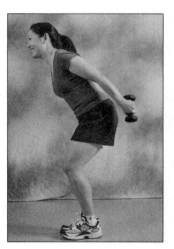

2. **Triceps kickback:** Stand with a slight bend in the knees and a slight hinge forward from the waist. Keeping your elbows close to your sides, exhale as your arms extend behind your body. Bend your arms back in on the inhale and repeat.

Figures 6.25

Lateral raise.

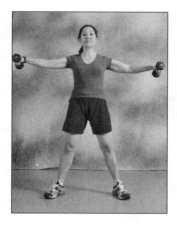

3. **Lateral raise:** Stand with your arms down by your sides. Lift your arms to the side, no higher than shoulder height while exhaling. Return your arms back down to your sides while inhaling and repeat.

Figures 6.26

Squats.

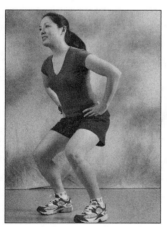

4. **Squats:** Stand with your legs hip width apart, abdominals tight, shoulders back, and chest lifted. Exhale while descending into a squat, as if sitting in a chair, keeping your weight centered over your heels. Make sure your knees do not go beyond your toes.

Figures 6.27

Lunges.

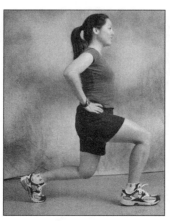

5. **Lunges:** Stand, feet together, and exhale, stepping one leg forward, bending both knees. Your back knee should remain parallel to the floor, while your front knee should not go beyond your toes. Keep your chest lifted and abdominals tight and strong.

Figures 6.28

Leg lifts.

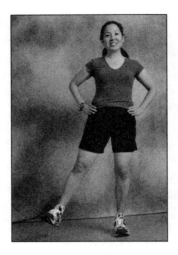

6. **Leg lifts:** Stand with your feet together, abdominals tight, shoulders back, and chest lifted. Keep your toes pointing forward, lift one leg out to the side while exhaling, and return back to start position on the inhale. Try to avoid shifting your weight to one side and leaning into your supporting leg.

If you're looking for an exercise DVD that is a great workout, I recommend Physique 57 DVDs. The ballet-based workout is created from the famous New York City classes by Tanya Becker. It's also a great workout for men.

Discharge Care Plan

For fun, to be formally discharged from this chapter please use your prioritizing nursing skill to reinforce some of the key messages of the chapter. Place what you think would be the correct prioritized number 1-4 in order of importance next to the corresponding letter.

A. __ Assertively schedule fitness into your daily lifestyle.

B. __ Engage in fitness you enjoy.

C. __ I'm important enough to deserve to feel healthier by actively engaging in physical activity.

D. __ Whenever I feel the urge to exercise, I lie down and let it pass.

Congratulations! You have earned a Golden Nightingale Wellness Wing by completing the interactive portions of the chapter!

(A = 3; B = 2; C = 1; D = 4)

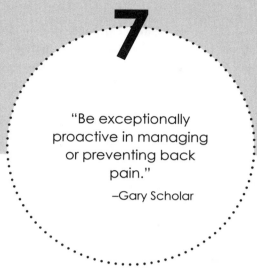

7

"Be exceptionally proactive in managing or preventing back pain."

–Gary Scholar

Taking Back Your Back: Reducing or Eliminating Your Back Pain Through Lifestyle and Fitness

–Karen Remond, MS, CHEK Certified,
CHEK* Faculty, Corrective, Exercise Specialist,
Holistic Health and Lifestyle Coach

–Caroline Jung, LAc, MSOM Certified Acupuncturist,
Master of Science in Oriental Medicine

–Gary Scholar, M.Ed.

Corrective Holistic Exercise Kinesiology

An estimated 52% of nurses complain of chronic back pain because of repeated lifting, transferring, and repositioning of patients throughout their working lifetime (American Nurses Association, 2005). In this chapter two highly regarded wellness professionals examine proactive measures on how to treat back pain.

●●●●●EMPOWERING NURSES

"I do not know a nurse who hasn't had back pain. Regular exercise and weight lifting has made my back pain nonexistent now. Weights really help. They make your muscles stronger so it is harder to strain them."

–Allison, hospital nurse

"I did indeed experience back and neck pain. I have had epidurals and physical therapy, which have helped tremendously. I try to stretch morning and night (before and after work). I walk instead of run (whether on a treadmill or bike path). Walking is great for the cardio and does limber one up. It's most important to stretch before and after. I find running to hurt my low back and knees."

–Renee, resource nurse

"I have a lower back sore spot that flares up every year or so if I have not kept up with stretching and crunches. In the last few years, it has flared up every 6 months or more. Rest, NSAIDS, muscle relaxants, and heat for a few days takes care of it, but it is a terrible inconvenience and worry each time."

–Mara, hospital nurse

"I treated my back pain with stretching and a chiropractor."
–Linda, nurse and operating room team leader

"I had back pain for many years but had a lamenectomy about 20 years ago and have not had a problem since."

–Chuck, hospital nurse

The high rate of chronic back pain in nurses can largely be attributed to lifting and repositioning patients, leaning over patients to take readings and administer IV meds, and improper ergonomics when sitting at nurses' stations.

Factor that in with the added abdominal weight many nurses—along with the general population—carry due to unhealthy diet and lack of exercise, and you have the RX for too much stress on the back. This chapter will give you insightful wellness expertise on how to prevent or manage your chronic back pain.

LIVEWELL

"Every extra pound that's carried on your belly puts 5 to 10 pounds of pressure on your spine."

–Dr. Mark McLaughlin, spine specialist

Personal Experience with Back Pain

Not only do I understand the epidemic of chronic back pain among nurses from a professional standpoint, I myself have suffered from it. I share my experiences with you in the hope I can help a number of nurses with the experience I went through. My back pain was due to the many years of contact sports. A number of years ago I started experiencing numbness in my toes on my left foot. Believing it was due to the wrong athletic shoes, I continued playing sports. Later, I began to feel a constant pain in my calf that felt like someone was hitting it with a sledgehammer. The pain was running from my knee to my foot. An MRI confirmed I had lumbar stenosis and disk herniation on a nerve root. I had two epidurals and ended up having lamenectomy and microdisketomy surgery.

I stopped contact sports, but played tennis and golf for 3 more years. Then I experienced pain again, and the MRI revealed two slightly bulging discs above where I had the surgery before, which can happen because in some cases after surgery your back is more vulnerable if you are not taking care of it properly.

I was determined to find a treatment that would help me manage my chronic pain. I wanted to not just relieve the pain but to incorporate lifestyle changes that would help me for the rest of my life. This is when I started working with Karen Redmond, MS, CHEK certified, corrective exercise specialist, and holistic health and lifestyle coach. With the help of her professional expertise, I am now performing daily back exercises and stretches that strengthen my core, and I have incorporated weight training as well. Redmond has encouraged me to change many aspects of my lifestyle that places me in the best possible mechanics, alignment, and posture to support my back—from proper back and sitting support while driving my car to proper mechanics in lifting and carrying—and even to brushing my teeth. In fact, I typed this book while sitting on a Swiss Ball (also sometimes called an exercise ball)! This places me in proper alignment and strengthens my core at the same time. The result is I'm back to playing tennis and golf, as well as back to my daily walking program. I have the tools to help me the rest of my life. I also have incorporated acupuncture and massage. Tai Chi, Pilates, and yoga can also be helpful. All of these changes are not just treatments for my back, but lifestyle changes as well.

A Note About Massage Therapy

Not only can massage help alleviate back pain, but it is also one of the most effective wellness services offered—particularly important for the success of a nurse's well-being. If you are a Nurse Type E personality (refer back to Chapter 3 for a discussion of Nurse Type E personalities) and you are doing everything for everyone but yourself, a massage is the one time that you can let go and let someone else take care of you. It might be one of the only opportunities in your professional and personal life that the activity is all about you. Not only does it feel wonderful, but it can also serve as an important learning tool to place self care as a priority in your life.

If you are considering creating a wellness program for nurses in your facility, massage is one of the first wellness services you should consider offering—even if only 10-minute chair massages during work hours. For example, a number of years ago I placed a pilot wellness program that offered massage therapy for nurses into Children's Memorial Hospital in Chicago, Illinois. Since then, Children's Memorial Hospital has created the Caring for the Caregiver Therapeutic Massage Program under the leadership of massage therapist Michelle Johnson that allows participating staff to receive 10 minute chair massages within their units structured around their breaks and lunch. The program is so successful they have a participation rate of 80% throughout the hospital.

Maia Bielak, a licensed massage therapist for the employees of the American Hospital Association and a massage therapist for my pilot program for nurses, explains the benefits of massage for nurses with back or other forms of pain and stress:

> Human touch is imperative to our survival, healing, and growth. Therefore, massage can provide nurses with increased energy needed for their demanding schedules, and a better understanding of how touch affects both the receiver and giver. The physical benefits for your

back pain are wonderful. As your body relaxes, blood pressure lowers, cells are stimulated to release toxins, and the entire nervous system is affected including the area that is causing your back pain. Specific back pain issues can be addressed and alleviated or even eliminated with massage, over time, if the back pain is not extremely severe. Chronic back pain can also create stress. Massage reconnects the mind with the body, a connection that is often lost in times of stress caused or exacerbated by back pain.

There are many helpful ways a therapist might treat low/lumbar back pain. Many therapists might begin with some basic clinical testing to determine or rule out certain aspects. To treat basic low/ lumbar back pain, the therapist might begin with hydrotherapy and myofascial release for the muscles of the low back, side body, and gluteals. He or she might address, with a variety of techniques, the origins, insertions, and bellies of the muscles in the aforementioned areas, working deeper into the mulifidi, the tiny muscles that run up and down the spine, and finally ending with stretching of the side body, low back, gluteals, hips, hamstrings, and quadriceps.

A Note About Back Pain and Your Feet

Because of the demanding amount of time nurses spend on their feet it is important to identify how your feet can affect your back pain. Dr. Max Barret of North Shore Physical Wellness explains, "Weaknesses or imbalances in your feet can affect your spine. When you spend a lot of time standing or walking as a nurse, your body is subjected to natural forces and postures that can stress and strain up your body's kinetic chain to your spine." Custom molded orthotics can help address back pain and provide support with each step. They should be flexible, custom-made orthotics that you wear in your shoes as these will support all three arches of your foot. Exact measurements of your feet should be taken, preferably from a digital foot scan.

The Usual Disclaimer

As a reminder, it is important to discuss introducing an exercise program into your back pain management regime with your care provider. If any exercise causes pain, you should discontinue it immediately.

More Than Just the Movement—Lifestyle and Back Pain

Back pain can affect the quality of your life including daily activities and work. Back pain is often not specifically diagnosed, making it difficult for treatment. In understanding how to manage back pain, you need to address the following points:

- **Nutrition:** You need a diet that is rich in anti-inflammatory foods that supports the immune system and healing of the musculoskeletal system.

- **Inflammatory foods that should be avoided:** Grains that contain gluten (wheat, barley, hops, rye, bulgur, couscous, kamut, matzo, and spelt), soy, white potatoes, sugar, fried foods, night shade vegetables (white potatoes, eggplant, tomatoes, bell peppers), sugar, artificial sweeteners.

- **Anti-inflammatory foods:** Wild caught salmon, halibut, sardines, cod, coconut, organic meats, organic whole eggs, and vegetables.

- **Hydration:** Drink one-half your body weight in ounces of water. For example, if you weigh 150 pounds, you should drink 75 ounces of water. You cannot count sodas or other carbonated beverages (except seltzer water), coffees, or caffeinated teas. You can include soup broth and herbal teas. Water should be free of chemicals and additives, preferably from a clean spring source, and should ideally contain 300 ppm (parts per million) of dissolved solids (that is, trace minerals that are naturally occurring in the water.)

- **Stress:** Personal and work

- **Ergonomics:** In home and office

- **Lifting mechanics**

- **Sleep**

- **Exercise**

- **Weight management**

Acute or Chronic: Identifying Symptoms and Referral to a Health Care Practitioner

You need to identify the type of pain:

- **Acute:** Onset of pain is quick, severe, and often occurs after a specific injury. Anyone with acute pain should seek professional medical attention immediately.

- **Chronic:** Pain or discomfort that persists or progresses over a period of time. This pain is often harder to categorize when it persists over a long period because it cannot always be linked to one specific event. Rather, it is typically cumulative.

Orthopedic Injuries

You should see an orthopedist, chiropractor, physical therapist, or CHEK practitioner. Medical imaging might be necessary.

Spinal Stenosis

Spinal stenosis is the narrowing of the vertebral canal. Space encroached by vertebrae does not allow ideal space for the nerves. Space left in the vertebral canal becomes too small, relatively, for the volume of nerves it has to transmit (Bogduk, 1997). This condition can be congenital or a result of poor posture and movement patterns, disease, or degeneration.

Symptoms include bilateral pain in back, buttocks, thighs, calves, and feet. It affects more men and involves insidious pain.

Activities that increase pain are extension, rotation, side bending, and walking. Activities that decrease pain are flexion, sitting, and prolonged rest.

Spondylolisthesis

Defects in the posterior elements, notably the pars interarticularis fractures, threaten to allow the vertebrae to slip progressively forward (Bogduk, 1997). Commonly found around age 20.

Symptoms include: back pain, insidious.

Activities that increase pain include standing, bending, rotation, and extension. Activities that decrease pain include sitting and lying down.

Commonly found at L5/S1.

Disc Pain

Symptoms include the following:

- Usually one-sided pain

- Sharp or shooting pain that refers

- Pain worse in morning

- Pain might present with a "shift," where the shoulders are going the opposite direction from the pelvis.

Activities that increase disc pain include axial loading, forward flexion, rotation, side bending, sitting, prolonged standing, sneezing, coughing, and bowel movements. Activities that decrease pain include lying supine, extension, and decompression.

Clinical Instability

Clinical instability is a condition in which any movement, small or large, causes a displacement or shifting of the vertebrae due to a lack of stability in the spine. It is often described as a vulnerable feeling, as if movement would cause the spine to stiffen up or lock down. If the segment is not "stabilized" optimally during movement (movement control), then the vertebrae shifts or becomes misaligned (Bogduk, 1997).

Symptoms include the following: Local back pain, might refer to vulnerable feeling; chronic ache or ache with particular movements; tenderness to palpation at vertebral points. Pain might be worse in morning or worse at end of day (or both).

Activities that increase pain include excessive ranges of movement (flexion, extension, rotation, and side bending) and quick or unexpected jerky movements. Activities that decrease pain include neutral spine, stable movement, and sometimes lying supine.

Sacroiliac Joint Pain

Sacroiliac joint (SIJ) pain might occur by itself or in conjunction with any of the above mentioned orthopedic issues. Pain might be one sided on the posterior superior iliac spine (PSIS) or across the entire SIJ. SIJ pain might also refer to the hip or glute area.

Pain usually occurs with movement; however, it might also occur when you are seated or standing. The pain might also change. Lying might relieve the pain. A compression hip belt (SIJ belt) might relieve the pain. Pain can be intermittent or chronic. A self or assisted SIJ mobilization (a manual therapy technique performed on joints that do not have normal range of motion) is often helpful in managing the pain by aligning the pelvis.

An Integrated Approach to Managing Back Pain

After you have discovered the pain generator, then a treatment/management plan should be formulated. You need to decide who is going to design your program. You need a chiropractor, physical therapist, or CHEK Practitioner Level II or higher to do this. Your program should comprise the following steps:

Step 1

Reduction of pain:

- Avoidance of provocative movement
- Moving and exercising in proper form
- Correct ergonomics
- Rest, ice, sleep
- Nutrition
- Adequate hydration
- Corrective stretches and exercises
- Therapy

Step 2

After the pain has been managed, the next step is to address the origin of the pain. Just because the pain has gone does not mean that you have addressed the reason why it occurred in the first place. To prevent a recurrence, you must stabilize and strengthen the muscles that support the lumbar spine and sacroiliac joint. These muscles include the spinal stabilizers: multifidus, transversus abdominis (TVA), and pelvic floor muscles. Each of these spinal stabilizers needs to be independently tested by a practitioner to determine if the muscles there have a proper recruitment pattern and optimal strength.

The abdominal canister contains the pelvis, five vertebrae of the lumbar spine, the lower six thoracic segments, and all the muscles that support these areas (deep and superficial muscle systems). A total of 85 joints must be supported and controlled (Lee, 2008). The attention to all these areas is critical. In the past, health professionals have focused primarily on the lumbar spine in diagnosis and treatment. The relationship between the lumbar spine, pelvis, and thoracic spine must be evaluated and treated. An injury, improper movement pattern, poor posture, weak muscles, and/or faulty muscle recruitment patterns can disrupt the proper function of the abdominal canister, so paying attention to all these areas is the key to recovery. Instead of isolating therapy on just the symptom, an integrated approach of looking at the function of the abdominal canister is crucial in restoring function to the body and preventing recurrence of an injury.

Stabilization precedes force generation (work); therefore, you need to make sure these muscles work properly before movement occurs. If you don't make sure those muscles work properly, you can think of yourself as a race car driving fast with loose lug nuts on the tires. Such a race car does not drive steadily and might even crash.

Other muscles that need to be strengthened include the following: latissimus dorsi; gluteus maximus, medius, and minimus; illiopsoas; lumbar erectors; quadriceps and biceps femoris. These muscles should be strengthened using functional integrated exercises in cooperation with the stabilizer muscles. Isolation exercises should be used only in acute situations or if the functional exercises cannot be performed. One of the major flaws in conventional rehabilitation exercises is the failure to progress from static and floor-based exercises to dynamic functional exercises that require dynamic control of the spine and pelvis. It is ideal in the management of people with low back pain to retrain dynamic control of the spine and pelvis during movement (Hodges & Cholewicki, 2007). This involves developing movement control strategies.

The following should be measured and evaluated:

- Muscular length tension imbalances
- Postural imbalances
- Nerve root tension
- Joint mobility and stability
- Sacroiliac joint mobility, alignment, and stability
- Functional movement pattern assessment that addresses work, life, and sport movements and activities

A CHEK Practitioner Level II or higher, physical therapist, or chiropractor can help to develop a program using the findings just mentioned.

The program should contain the following:

- Corrective stretches and joint mobilizations to address postural musculoskeletal imbalances
- Stabilization exercises using a Swiss Ball and/or done on the floor
- Neuromuscular isolation exercises (multifidus, TVA, and pelvic floor) when needed
- Functional dynamic movements that carry over to daily life activities, work, and sport

Step 3

Re-evaluation, increased strength, and progression of program to make you stronger.

Step 4

Re-evaluation, maintenance exercises, stretches, and follow-up with practitioner.

Other Resources

Massage therapy and acupuncture are great resources in helping to manage pain and heal injuries.

Ergonomics

Ergonomics ensure that you are maintaining proper posture and alignment. Poor posture can create or exacerbate an injury or pain.

Your computer monitor should be positioned so that when you are sitting in good posture—knees bent at a 90-degree angle, back and neck straight—the center of the computer screen is aligned with the center of your eye. The keyboard needs to be at a height that puts the elbows at 90 degrees with the wrists supported. Feet should be flat on the floor. One option is to sit on a Swiss Ball at your desk; this allows your body to be in a more ideal postural position. Another option is a standing desk. If you use a laptop, keep it on a laptop stand and use a wireless mouse and wireless keyboard.

Sleeping

Sleep is one of the most important parts of the day. During sleep, the body heals at both the neurological and cellular levels. It is important to not only get enough sleep (7-8 hours of uninterrupted sleep), but to try to sleep between 10 pm and 6 am. When you go to bed at 10pm, melatonin, which works as a powerful antioxidant helps to repair damage in the body.

- It is important to sleep with your spine and pelvis in a neutral position, which minimizes compression and torsion. If you do not sleep this way, then you may exacerbate your condition.

- Sleep lying with your hips flexed to 90 degrees and a pillow between your knees, or sleep lying on your back with your knees bent and a pillow or bolster under the knees.

Strengthening the Core and the Back

Strengthening the core and back muscles is critical in maintaining optimal spine and pelvis alignment (neutral spine). Exercising in neutral spine will teach movement control which stabilizes the spine. This will allow the body to move in a pain-free zone. This is important to be able to resume work and life activities without pain.

Self Trigger Point Massage on the Hip and Gluteal Muscles

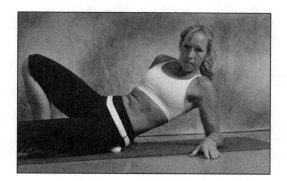

Figure 7.1

Self trigger point massage on the hip and gluteal muscles.

Self releasing of trigger points in the hip and gluteal area is an important component to pain management. A trigger point is an area within the muscle that hyperirritable and when compressed is tender and may cause referred pain to other areas such as joints or organs (Travell and Simons, 1983). Where trigger points exist, the tissue is ischemic (blood flow is diminished to the area). This reduces the capacity of the muscle to work. Painful trigger points may also cause muscles to shut down by going into a protective mode. Many people have weak glute muscles and in order to maximize muscle function, the trigger points must be released and circulation improved. An increase of blood flow to the affected area will bring nutrients to heal the tissue. Lie on your side with a tennis ball under your hip. Roll around on the tennis ball. When you find a tender spot (trigger point), roll back and forth over that area. Make sure you move the ball around the entire hip area to find all the trigger points.

Four-Point Transversus Abdominis Activation Trainer: How to Find Your Neutral Spine

Figure 7.2

In neutral position, the pole should touch the back of the head, between the shoulder blades and at the sacrum.

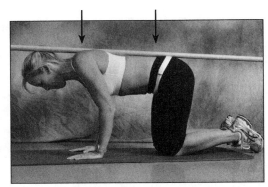

Photo is based upon image from The Golf Biomechanic's Manual *by Paul Chek. Published by the C.H.E.K Institute in 2001.*

When you are in the four-point position as shown in Figure 7.2, place a pole in the center of the back from the head down to the sacrum. The pole should be 6 feet long and approximately 1 1/4 to 1 1/2 inches in diameter. A wooden closet dowel rod works well. The pole should touch the back of the head, between the shoulder blades and the sacrum. The pole should not touch your lower back; you should have a gap between the lumbar spine and the pole. The ideal space is approximately the size of the thickest part of your hand between your back and the pole. Neutral spine should be "pain-free." Depending on varying spinal pathologies, some people need less lumbar curve. For example, someone with severe stenosis or a spondylolisthesis will find that their neutral spine is very flat. In this case, the flatter lumbar curve relieves pain by opening up the foramen in the spine. This neutral position might feel a little foreign, but it should not cause pain. Keep in mind that holding neutral spine can be very fatiguing to muscles, and you might experience mild muscular soreness.

Maintaining a neutral spine during movement is essential in retraining the body to move without causing injury. Many injuries are caused by moving and lifting in poor posture and poor alignment repeatedly. You should be evaluated before returning to movements, lifting in flexion, or with lumbar kyphosis. The body should be ideally strengthened, and you should be free of pain. This activity should be done under supervision to ensure it is safe.

Your hands should be under your shoulders, and your hips should be at 90 degrees. Completely relax your abdominals, making sure you have no muscle tone. Using a full diaphragmatic breath, inhale and the belly and ribcage should expand; exhale gently through pursed lips and draw the belly button gently up like you are trying to get it to touch your spine (do not exhale completely). This is activating your TVA. Hold this and count to 10 out loud.

Exercise	Repetitions	Time	Sets	Rest
Four-Point TVA Trainer	10 per set	10 sec hold	1–3	1 minute

You should do this daily for the first 1–3 weeks for neuromuscular reprogramming of your abdominal wall (Chek, 1999).

Four-Point Transversus Abdominis Activation Trainer: Lifting from the Floor

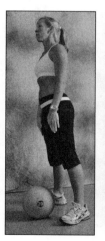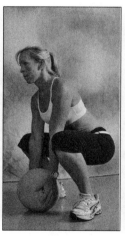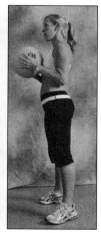

Figure 7.3

You can use a basketball-size ball or simply imagine you are lifting something.

Standing upright with your feet slightly wider than your hips, gently activate your TVA as before (completely relax your abdominals, making sure you have no muscle tone and take a full diaphragmatic breath—inhale and expand the belly and ribcage—and exhale through pursed lips while gently drawing in the belly button like you are trying to get it to touch your spine (do not exhale completely). Bend your knees and stick your butt back as you lower to a squat with your butt near your heels, being careful to maintain a neutral spine at all times. Push up through your heels when you stand up. Count to 10 while you do the lift.

DonTigny Seated Knee Reach Sacroiliac Joint Mobilization

This mobilization helps to align the SIJ. Sit in a firm chair or on a stool in good posture with your feet flat. Put pressure into your right heel and push your right knee forward so that it moves slightly ahead of the left, while pulling your left knee back toward your body. These actions should be done simultaneously. Hold this for 3–5 seconds and repeat several times, alternating each side. This mobilization can also be done lying on your back on the floor. You can do this a few times per hour throughout the day (DonTigny, 1994).

Horse Stance

Figure 7.4

Horse stance.

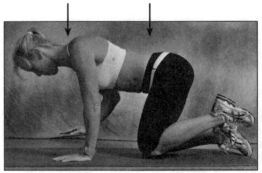

Get on the floor on four points, just as you did for the activity with Figure 7.2 to find your neutral spine and activate your TVA. Make sure that your spine is neutral. Activate your TVA as before. Lift your right hand and your left knee off the floor about half an inch and hold. Then perform with the left hand and right knee lifting off the floor. Your spine should remain neutral, and you should have no rotation, side bending, or leaning to the side.

Exercise	Repetitions	Time	Sets	Rest
Horse Stance	6–10 each side per set	hold each 5–10 sec	1–2	1 minute

Swiss Ball Hip Extension Feet on Floor

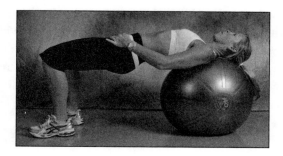

Figure 7.5

Swiss Ball hip extension with feet on the floor.

Roll out on the Swiss Ball on your back. Your head and shoulder blades should be supported on the ball. Your feet and ankles should be directly under the knees (90 degrees). Lift your hips up and focus on squeezing your gluteus maximus, gluteus medius, and gluteus minimus. All your glute muscles should be firm to the touch. Be careful not to overbridge (lifting up too high) by using your spinal erector muscles (low back muscles). You can also do this holding onto the frame in a doorway for additional stability.

Exercise	Repetitions	Time	Sets	Rest
Swiss Ball Hip Extension Feet on Floor	6–10	hold each 5–10 sec	1–3	1 minute

Swiss Ball Seated Posture Trainer

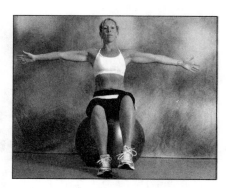

Figure 7.6

Swiss Ball seated posture trainer.

Swiss Ball Seated Posture Trainer photo is based upon the image from Equal, But Not the Same *correspondence course manual by Paul Chek. Published by the C.H.E.K Institute 1998-2008.*

Sit on Swiss Ball in front of a mirror. Sit up tall with good posture. Maintain a neutral lumbar spine by slightly rolling your pelvis forward. Your chest should be lifted, ears in line with your shoulders, and your feet should be in alignment directly under your knees with approximately 2–4 inches between the feet. At all times in the exercise keep your shoulders and hips parallel to each other and square to the mirror (no rotation in hips or trunk). Extend your arms to the side and lift one foot a few inches off the floor. You should have little to no movement of the ball (Chek, 1998-2008).

Exercise	Repetitions	Time	Sets	Rest
Swiss Ball Seated Posture Trainer	3–6 each side	hold each 5–10 sec	1–2	1:00

Forward Ball Roll

Figure 7.7

Forward ball roll.

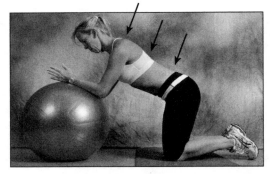

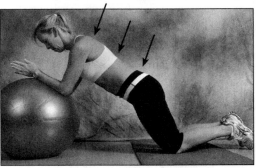

Photo is based upon image from The Golf Biomechanic's Manual *by Paul Chek. Published by the C.H.E.K Institute 2001.*

Kneel on the floor with your forearms on the ball, like you are praying. Your spine should be neutral, your eyes focused on your hands. Activate your TVA. Hold that activation and roll forward without moving your knees. Your hips and arms should move synchronously. Roll forward a few inches and hold for 5–10 seconds. Keeping your TVA activation, roll back to the start and relax. Repeat. Do each repetition with a complete re-setting of your TVA (Chek, 2001).

Exercise	Repetitions	Time	Sets	Rest
Forward Ball Roll	6–8	hold 5–10 sec	1–2	1:00

Traditional Chinese Medicine (TCM): Treatment and Prevention

Acupuncture is an effective therapy to use for back pain because it frees up any stagnant energy in the body that may cause pain. Or if you have a deficiency of energy along a meridian, then the acupuncture supplements this area and relieves the pain. One of the wonderful aspects of TCM is that it can be safely used in conjunction with other types of therapy. Many of my patients who come in with pain are also seeing a physical therapist or chiropractor to help reduce their symptoms. Acupuncture and other TCM modalities can be used at the same time as Western medicine therapies. TCM can actually enhance the effects of other therapies in a positive way.

Acupuncture— The insertion of fine, thin, sterile needles into points (the acupuncture points) along the meridians of the body to balance the *qi* (pronounced *chi* or *chee*.)

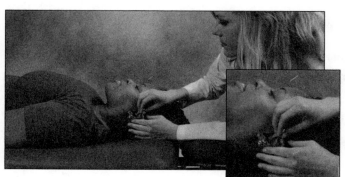

Figure 7.8

Inserting an acupuncture needle in the ear.

Figure 7.9

Cupping.

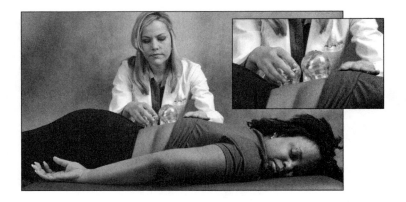

Treatment for Back Pain

TCM practitioners look at your whole body, including the mind and spirit when forming your diagnosis. In general, we understand that pain is caused by a stagnation or deficiency of your qi. This pain can present itself as a sharp or dull pain and/or a localized or wandering pain. For example, if your qi is stagnant in your lower back, then it is likely you are going to have pain in your back. The same is true of deficiency as well. If your qi is insufficient along a meridian, you might experience a type of dull pain or discomfort along that meridian or surrounding area. As an example, low back pain is associated with a deficiency along your kidney meridian. A reason for this is a natural decline of your "yin" energy. You are born with a certain amount of both yin and yang. Both aspects slowly decline as you age. The yin and yang of your body can be more easily depleted from excessive stress, inadequate exercise, and also inadequate rest and sleep. In TCM we look closely at your sleep patterns, digestion, bowel movements, appetite, diet, stress and energy levels, predominant emotions, and menstrual cycles for women; all of this tells us what is going on in your entire body. We also use palpation along different areas of your body and your meridians to see where you might have more tenderness, which represents a qi stagnation or deficiency.

Cupping—A therapy in which a cupping jar is placed over a flat area of the body to create a partial vacuum over the skin, usually by introducing heat from a flame.

Along with the general physical demands of being a nurse, if you have any excess heat or cold in the body, it can compound pain. This pain can, in turn, disrupt your sleep pattern, which makes your workday even more challenging because of your fatigue. Your yin energy is active at night, so if you are getting inadequate sleep, your back pain might be exacerbated. Depending on your diagnosis, we can use many TCM therapies to treat your back pain. I usually begin with an acupuncture treatment combined with an herbal recommendation, although sometimes I use only the cupping therapy or only the gua sha therapy. Both of these are strong treatments that move a lot of energy, so patients see great results. I also integrate quick applications of tui na for pain; it is intense massage that can really move pain out of the body. The moxibustion is a really nice therapy I use with my patients who might be nervous about the needles. With TCM we can use any combination of these therapies or use them alone. The balanced harmonious flow of your qi is what decreases any pain.

Back pain might also stem from stress and/or tension. Meditation and relaxation are two key components to releasing tension in the body.

The number and duration of treatments differ for each patient. The longer you have had a symptom, the longer it might take for it to completely dissipate. After your symptoms have diminished, I recommend using TCM as a preventive medicine. For example, most patients with sciatica tend to have a flare up once a year or for some nurses it might be a few times a year. It varies from individual to individual, but using acupuncture and herbs to keep your qi balanced can help prevent the symptoms from returning. Also, if your symptoms do return, they tend to be less severe.

Moxibustion—A form of therapy using Chinese herbs that are heated and burned over the acupuncture points.

Tui na—Tui na (pronounced *thway na*) is a form of Chinese deep tissue massage.

Chinese Herbs—Single herbs or formulas of herbs used to treat illnesses—taken in raw herb tea form, pills, tinctures, or powders.

Gua sha—A type of therapy using a "gua sha" (pronounced *gwa shaw*) tool, which looks like a ceramic spoon, to scrape and rub an area of the body to balance the qi.

Discharge Care Plan

For fun, to be formally discharged from this chapter please use your prioritizing nursing skills to reinforce some of the key messages of the chapter. Place what you think would be the correct prioritized number 1-9 in importance next to the corresponding letter.

A. __ Pain usually stems from a stagnation or deficiency that can be alleviated without side effects using TCM.

B. __ Meditation combined with TCM is a powerful tool to help mange chronic back pain.

Finding Fitness

TCM to Help With Chronic Lower Back Pain

Laura, a nurse, is 38 years old, has three children, and was an ER nurse before becoming a nurse midwife. Laura had chronic back pain for the last 2 years. On a scale of 1–10, her pain was usually around 5. She did not have any history of back pain or injury. She reported her back pain decreased when she went to her weekly yoga class. After a complete exam, my diagnosis was that Laura had qi deficiency and kidney yin deficiency. The qi deficiency, I believed, stemmed from the physical and emotional demands of her job. It could also have been from her duties as a mother—taking care of her family, household responsibilities, and so on. The kidney yin deficiency is associated with the low back pain. In addition, the kidney yin deficiency was probably also associated with perimenopause, because it is one of the energies in your body that begins to decline and is more apparent when menopause and perimenopause begins.

My recommendation for Laura was to use acupuncture 2 times a week for about 4 weeks. After the second week, her back pain was at a 2 out of 10. After that, I recommended she come in 2 times the next week and then start coming once a week. I did use cupping along with the acupuncture during a few of the treatments. I also recommended an herbal formula for Laura to help alleviate the night sweats she was experiencing. This situation serves as an example of how we can treat more than one symptom at a time with TCM. After 3 months of treatment, I recommended she come in 2 times a month to prevent the low back pain from flaring up again.

I believe that our bodies are constantly striving to remain in homeostasis and that our bodies can take and apply whatever tools and therapies we give it to stay healthy. TCM is effective and gentle at the same time.

C. __ TCM integrates your entire body systems and what is going on in your life to make an effective diagnosis and treatment plan.

D. __ An integrated approach is the most effective treatment. It includes stress management, ergonomics, lifting mechanics, sleep, exercise, weight management, nutrition, hydration, and avoidance of provocative movement.

E. __ Identifying the symptoms and type of pain is the first step in treating your back pain.

F. __ Scheduling an MRI is an important tool for diagnosis.

G. __ You need to treat the pain and also make positive changes in your lifestyle that can help keep that pain from becoming chronic in the future.

H. __ The massage therapist, chiropractor, physical therapist, orthopedic physician, and CHEK practitioner and all health care professionals can help treat your back pain.

I. __ Performing cartwheels down the hall of your hospital, office, or school is an effective preventive treatment for back pain, or more likely, it will land you in the hospital.

Congratulations! You have earned a Golden Nightingale Wellness Wing by completing the interactive portions of the chapter!

(A = 1; B = 1; C = 1; D = 1; E = 1; F = 1; G. = 1; H = 1) (Okay, don't be upset, but all of the messages are too important to prioritize, not counting I, of course!)

"Healthy eating is a wonderful act of self kindness!"

–Gary Scholar

Getting Out of Your Comfort Zone:
Recognizing the Signs and Changing the Behaviors of Comfort Eating

Many years ago I found myself standing in the frozen food section flirting with the prospect of buying a mouth-watering strawberry cheesecake. I rationalized buying it by convincing myself I would eat only one small piece. So there I was later, being a couch potato and watching T.V. when I gave in to my craving and made a beeline to my dear friend the refrigerator. I plopped the frozen cheesecake on my lap in front of the TV and, without giving the dessert a chance to thaw out, I transformed in an instant from Dr. Jekyll to Mr. Hyde and devoured the entire thing. I unconsciously wolfed down the *entire* cheesecake within minutes! (It must have been a full moon.) That, my dear nurses, is a classic example of comfort binge eating.

Looking back, I realized I was looking for satisfaction; that is, I was eating that night to find comfort for four distinct reasons:

1. The first reason had nothing to do with food, but everything to do with trying to fill an emotional need. I was bored! What I've learned about myself since is that boredom is the number one reason I comfort eat.

2. Location: I had easy access to the cheesecake in the refrigerator.

3. The way I ate back then created a negative roller-coaster effect with my blood sugar level. When it dropped low, it triggered my craving for comfort food.

4. The fourth reason, let's be honest. I love cheesecake!

I share my comfort food story with you because I know for many nurses comfort eating presents a difficult challenge to eating healthier, managing their weight, and maintaining their energy level.

Discomfort Food

"Comfort food"—donuts, cookies, cakes, starchy vegetables, fatty meats, fried foods, and various other "comforts"—is everywhere in your work environment, and likely in your home environment and at every family and social gathering. You are tempted at the nurses' station, break room, vending machines, and hospital cafeterias. If that's not enough, you might decide to drive through a fast food restaurant on the way home because you are so exhausted. And, of course, you likely have some comfort food waiting for you at home.

Examining Nurse Comfort Eating

You might comfort eat for a variety of emotional reasons; you might feel stress caused by your work environment, home life, relationships, finances, health, or you might feel exhausted, bored, lonely, anxious, frustrated, overwhelmed, or depressed. Comfort foods seem like they can be a quick fix to help manage your looping, but then you compound it with the guilt associated with unhealthy eating or overeating. Comfort eating has a lot to do with satisfaction and can translate into how you manage your life. If your needs aren't being met successfully, sometimes food seems like an easy option to make you feel better. There are three easy reasons that contribute to why we comfort eat:

1. Location, location, location.

2. SCRUBS (Sugar Cravings Ruin Blood Sugar)

3. Skipping meals

Feeding Frenzy

"When I was in the hospital, my daughter—bless her heart—brought in a huge basket of assorted chocolates for the nurses as a way to thank them for taking such great care of me. Honestly, it was as if there was a Code Chocolate sounding in the nurses' station. It seemed like every nurse stopped by my room. My room became central station for a feeding frenzy! But I think I got a little extra care because of it!"

–Edward, 78-year-old patient in the hospital recovering from hip replacement surgery

---

Location, Location, Location

The proximity or availability of comfort food can raise your temptation level. Comfort foods tend to be very accessible to a nurse in the work environment. It's like having an IV of snacks, sweets, and candy permanently attached to your arm. And of course, after being completely exhausted after work the last thing you feel like doing is making dinner. The location and accessibility of drive-in fast food restaurants represent a giant magnet, drawing you into them. Even if you make it past the gauntlet of burgers and fries, you arrive home after a long day of taking care of your patients' needs to reward yourself with opening your Pandora refrigerator box only to find more comfort food. We haven't even talked about when you have a family and you're the only one that's trying to eat healthy, but lying in wait are your kid's favorite potato chips!

●●●●●EMPOWERING NURSES

Take Back the Station

Recruit patients' families and others in helping keep you and your colleagues healthy. Here are a few ideas for keeping unhealthy foods out of sight and out of mind.

- Set an example by bringing in fresh fruits or vegetables for snacking once a week or every few shifts. If you need it, ask for donations from those who are snacking with you. Most people are happy to contribute, and your actions will be contagious. Before you know it, it will become a habit, and someone will be bringing in homemade hummus and rice crackers, trail mix, and couscous salad to go along with your vegetables.

- Post signs. Some families will read the signs posted around the units. Explain that in an effort to be healthy, the nurses ask that any thoughtful "thank you" gifts not include high calorie, low nutrient snacks or desserts. If it feels more comfortable, list diabetes as a reason to not bring in the bad stuff.

- Suggested donations could be vegetable trays, fresh or dried fruit, assorted raw nuts, and so on.

- Instead of tempting nurses with unhealthy snacks tempt them with a chair massage!

SCRUBS (Sugar Cravings Ruin Blood Sugar)

Secondly, roller-coaster fluctuations of your blood sugar levels trigger comfort food cravings for high-calorie, sweet, and unhealthy fatty foods—or SCRUBS (sugar cravings ruin blood sugar). One of the observations I made when I shadowed nurses is the inability for some nurses to maintain and manage healthy blood sugar levels throughout their shifts. Nurses have expressed their lack of energy and feelings of fatigue. I call this *nurse glycemia*—roller-coaster fluctuations in blood sugars occur when nurses skip meals because they believe they don't have enough time to eat. Skipping a meal triggers low blood sugar and causes overeating at the next meal. Also eating highly refined foods can raise your blood sugar level quickly and then drop it like a rock, which can also lead to overeating at the next meal.

Foods that create satisfied, comfortable feelings—typically those high in refined carbohydrates and sugars—signal your pancreas to overreact, releasing too much insulin, first spiking the blood sugar level, then causing it to plummet. When your insulin returns to its lower level, the craving starts in again, repeating the cycle. This kind of blood sugar roller coaster can cause a dysfunctional metabolism, hormonal imbalances, and weight gain, headaches, migraines, and more severe PMS and menopause symptoms. You can have a more difficult time managing stress since lower blood sugar negatively effects how your brain can handle even the smallest irritations.

> ## Going and Going and Going
>
> "I go from my clinic to the hospital at noon and do my patient rounds, so most of the time I miss my lunch, and then at 3:30 p.m. I'm starving! So I grab a bag of pretzels, chocolate chip cookies, or a handful of M & M's."
>
> –Carmen, clinical and hospital nurse

The best way to hop off the roller coaster and select a gentler carousel ride is to eat every 3 or 4 hours, even if it's just a healthy snack. The snacks should consist of healthy protein and complex carbs. If you find yourself in a situation at work were you don't have time to snack, make sure you are hydrated with plenty of water to keep your energy level up. Also make it a priority that when you do eat your regular meal it is made up of healthy protein, whole grains, and fruit or vegetables to help keep your blood sugar level from plummeting over the course of the time that you are not eating.

Another contributing factor to the blood sugar roller coaster is eating low-fat desserts that are often loaded with added sugar to increase the flavor. So make sure you read your food label and try to have only 6 grams or less per serving of sugar. You can also dress up your own desserts with healthy fruits and nuts. This isn't the only reason to watch out for unhealthy low-fat desserts. Your body responds to them by failing to turn off the signal that you have had enough.

So what if you don't want to break up with your comfort foods. Your comforting three or more cups of coffee makes your heart beat faster, pitter patter. A drive-in double cheeseburger is the best double date you ever had. Cozying up to a bag of crunchy potato chips in front of the TV is so romantic. Chocolate chip ice cream—you're over the moon in love! That's what comfort food does. It's the "gotcha" factor that gets you with the first bite.

"Your comfort food has you head over heels, or in some cases belly over toes, in love!"

●●●●●EMPOWERING NURSES

PMS Sabotage

Are you one of the women nurses who experience uncontrollable cravings for chocolate, sweets, ice cream, or salty foods the week (or two) before your period? This can play havoc with your weight management, healthy eating, and blood sugar level maintenance.

There's a whole host of research and studies out that point to diet, nutrition (including supplements), and exercise as the answer to mild to moderate cases of PMS. (Extreme dysmenorrhea should be investigated with your health care provider.) In addition, the Nurse's Study II has revealed that women with higher intake of calcium and vitamin D have fewer and less severe PMS symptoms (Querna, 2005). Here's a list of commonly accepted nutrition and lifestyle changes that may help PMS sufferers from Womenshealth.gov (U.S. Department of Health and Human Services, n.d.):

- Exercise regularly.
- Eat healthy foods, including healthy proteins, fruits, vegetables, and whole grains.
- Avoid salt, sugary foods, caffeine, and alcohol, especially when you are having PMS symptoms.
- Get enough sleep. Try to get 8 hours of sleep each night.
- Find healthy ways to cope with stress. Use your assertiveness training to make sure your needs are being met. Talk to your friends, exercise, or write in a journal.
- Don't smoke.
- I would also include:
- Drink plenty of filtered water.
- Reduce salt intake to minimize swelling.
- Avoid coffee, soft drinks, and alcohol.
- Eat smaller meals throughout the day.
- Engage in physical activity—raises serotonin and lowers cortisol levels. (WebMD, n.d.)

What makes you also fall so hard for your comfort food is the addictive nature of your comfort food of choice. With refined sugars, serotonin is quickly released in your brain and makes you feel good when you eat a donut, chocolate, white bagel, and so on. Your brain has a terrific memory, so if you have comfort food in the morning, it's going to remember it and ask for it in the afternoon and night. Your comfort food has you head over heels, or in some cases belly over toes, in love!

Soft Drinks

The Nurses' Health Study Annual Newsletter, 2005, reported that soft drinks are the main source of added sugar in the nurse's diet that can contribute to weight gain. It found that over an 8-year period nurses gained an average of 17 pounds if they started drinking at least one sugar sweetened soft drink per day. In addition daily consumption of these beverages nearly doubled the risk of diabetes.

So what do you do if you want to change your lifestyle and eat healthier, besides giving up your job and staying at a secluded health spa for the rest of your life?

"Discharge" Comfort Food Intake

To eat healthier you first need to identify your top five comfort foods:

1. _____
   _____
   _____

2. _____
   _____
   _____

3. _____
   _____
   _____

4. _____
   _____
   _____

5. _____
   _____
   _____

Identify your top two emotional comfort food triggers (relationship, boredom, and so on):

1. _____

_____

_____

2. _____

_____

_____

Identify three of the most accessible locations of your comfort foods that can sabotage your efforts to eat healthier (nurses station, break room, home, and so on):

1. _____

_____

_____

2. _____

_____

_____

3. _____

_____

_____

You can help discharge your comfort foods by assertively taking the following proactive steps. You can implement assertiveness by making a paradigm shift in how you get your needs met. The following are some examples.

- If I'm bored, I structure my time. I read instead of watching so much TV. I knit, crochet, paint, or host a card game with my friends. I schedule time for tennis, biking, or take a nature walk with the kids.

- I spend quality time with my significant other.

- I schedule an honest talk with my spouse about making a commitment at any time to place needs on the table without the other person escalating or feeling defensive.

- I meet a like-minded potential love interest by being involved with a community service.

- I schedule a meeting with my supervisor to explain that I need to play more to my strengths when it comes to my job. This would not only benefit myself but benefit the entire staff.

- I request to work a different shift or floor that better suits my needs.

I W.I.N.—Is It What I Need?

For an easy reminder, make yourself a laminate bracelet with the letters IWIN. Every time you reach for an unhealthy comfort food it serves as a fun reminder—"Is It What I Need?" Do I really need to be assertive in getting my needs met or eating healthier comfort foods?

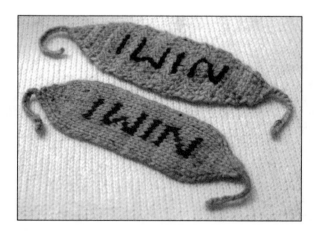

Figure 8.1

IWIN (Is It What I Need?) wrist bracelet.

I W.I.N.—I'm Worth It Now!

This meaning can remind you that you are worth making healthier food choices. You can create your own "I Win" wristlet, or you can knit the wristlet. Donna Palicka of Sister-Arts Studio in Chicago, created the knitting pattern.

Figure 8.2

IWIN (I'm Worth
It Now!) wrist
bracelet.

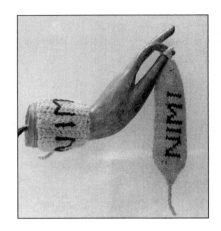

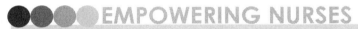
EMPOWERING NURSES

IWIN Knitting Pattern
"I WIN" knit wristlet:

Size:
Adult, one size fits all

Finished Dimensions:
12" long x 2 1/2" wide

Materials:
Any worsted weight yarn
2 colors: base and contrast color (cc)

Needles:
Size 7 or size to obtain gauge

Gauge:
5 1/4 stitches per inch

Pattern:
Cast-on 3 stitches with base color yarn

Rows 1, 3, 5, 7, and 9—Increase first and last stitch of each row for a total of 13 stitches

Rows 2, 4, 6, 8 &10—purl all stitches

Row 11—k4, k5 cc, k4 (letter I)

Row 12 and 14—p13

Row 13—k13

Row 15—k4, k5 cc, k4 (letter W)

Row 16—p8, p1 cc, p4

Row 17—k5, k1 cc, k7

Row 18—p6, p1 cc, p6

Row 19—k5, k1 cc, k7

Row 20—p8, p1 cc, p4

Row 21—k4, k5 cc, k4

Row 22—p13

Row 23—k13

Row 24—p4, p5 cc, p4 (letter I)

Row 25—k13

Row 26—p13

Row 27—k4, k5 cc, k4 (letter N)

Row 28—p4, p1 cc, p8

Row 29—k7, k1 cc, k5

Row 30—p6, p1 cc, p6

Row 31—k5, k1 cc, k7

Row 32—p8, p1 cc, p4

Row 33—k4, k5 cc, k4

Row 34—k13

Rows 35, 37, 39, 41, and 43—purl all stitches

Rows 36, 38, 40, 42, 44, and 46—decrease first and last stitch of each row until 1 stitch remains

Finishing

With crochet hook chain 12 stitches on the cast-on and bind and bind-of edges

Weave in ends

Block wristlet to lay flat

If you're not a knitter, you may be wondering what in the devil Gary Scholar is doing putting a knitting pattern in a wellness book. Well, the benefits of knitting are really what this book is all about. Knitting creates special self care time for nurses in which they are engaged in an activity that can relax them and give them a sense of satisfaction. Not unimportantly, it also keeps hands busy with purling and knitting instead of reaching for comfort food!

Finding Fitness

Rehabilitating Your Pantry

"Two years ago, when my daughter and I left the office of my surgeon, we could barely speak as the prognosis of my upcoming surgery wasn't very good, mostly because of my obesity. By the time we got home, my daughter had made up her mind that she was going to make sure I ate healthier. The following day she went through my pantry and cabinets and got rid of all the unhealthy foods I owned.

"After my kitchen was almost empty of food, we shopped for healthy, organic foods, and she taught me how to cook them . . . the daughter to the mom RN!!

"By the time of my surgery I had lost 30 lbs. After surgery, I cooked healthy and walked for exercise and lost an additional 35 lbs!"

–Carmen, clinical and hospital nurse

Some other strategies you can employ to discharge comfort foods involve dealing with location issues:

- Carry a "mobile munchy" snack (a handful of walnuts and almonds) at your nurses station or in your break room.

- Ask that unhealthy comfort food in the break room be placed in a "hidden" drawer or make a commitment to have a "comfort free food zone" in your nurses station/break room.

- Create a Code Brown "contamination" bin in your own kitchen by getting rid of your unhealthy comfort food.

Tossing out unhealthy foods in your kitchen makes you feel liberated because you feel more in control. Keeping your blood sugar stabilized and energy up throughout the day or night is critical care for nurses. Answer the following questions:

I feel at my best when:

- __ I read food labels and make sure what I buy has 6 grams of sugar or less per serving.

- __ Sugar, honey, high fructose corn syrup, dextrose, sucrose, or so on is the fourth ingredient or less on the food label.

- __ I try to reduce 5–10 grams of added sugar per day.

- __ I reduce or get rid of the amount of soft drinks, diet sodas, alcohol, and caffeine that spike my blood sugar.

___ I don't skip meals, which can cause a large drop in my blood sugar level.

___ I am consistent in the time and amount of food I consume each day.

___ I eat whole grains, lean proteins, legumes, vegetables, and fruit to produce a slow release of sugar because it takes more time to break down and be digested. Example:

- Breakfast: Egg whites and tomato omelet with a slice of whole grain bread and a glass of water

- Snack: Apple and almond butter

- Lunch: Avocado sandwich

- Snack: Rice crackers and hummus

- Dinner: Tilapia or a veggie burger, brown rice, and green salad

___ If I'm at a restaurant I do not eat the rolls or drink a soft drink before my order because if I do, by the time my order arrives my blood sugar has spiked and rapidly declined, causing me to eat more food then I intended to.

___ I stay off all added sugar for a month and see how much better I feel.

Diabetes and Nurses

The Nurses' Health Study Annual Newsletter, 2002, reports that some foods have what is called a high glycemic index, which means they can raise blood glucose rapidly. The study found that women nurses who ate the most high glycemic index foods had a 50% greater risk of diabetes than those who ate the least. Examples of high glycemic foods include baked white potatoes and white bread. Foods with a low glycemic index include apples, beans, and whole grain pasta.

Cutting Down Caffeine

If you try to reduce caffeine in your coffee too fast, you might experience headaches. Some cups of coffee have over 300 mg of caffeine. To deal with your coffee habit, consider the following:

"If you adopt only one assertive nutrition goal in this book, the comfort food exchange is the one."

1. Reduce amount of cups of coffee per day.

2. Try half of a cup of brewed and half decaf.

3. Try decaf, which has 3–5 mg of caffeine per cup.

So, how do you break up with your dysfunctional relationship with your beloved comfort food? You have to create a fulfilling relationship with new high-performance comfort food. You have to create a comfort food exchange. It's like breaking up with someone and the next day finding someone that is much better suited for you!

"Every time you go shopping, choose three or more new healthy foods you have never tried before in your life. Half the foods you try, you won't like, and you will never have again. But the other half you try, you will fall in love with. They will be your new comfort foods."

If you only adopt one assertive nutrition goal in this book, the comfort food exchange is the one. I did not enjoy food shopping before, but for many years now shopping for food is fun and exciting. It is the one thing that has completely changed how I eat. It's so simple, but the simplest things can be the most effective.

●●●●●●EMPOWERING NURSES

Shopping

You can choose from more than 55,000 food items in a typical grocery store. Every time you go shopping, choose three or more new healthy foods you have never tried before in your life. Half the foods you try, you won't like, and you will never have again. But the other half you try you will fall in love with. They will be your new comfort foods. No one said that comfort foods have to be unhealthy. Within a few months you have an entire new list of healthy comfort foods that you crave—in with the new, out with the old. I have stayed committed to shopping like this over many years, and I'm constantly finding new comfort foods I love. You won't ever get into a rut because you are bored with what you are eating if you are constantly trying new healthy foods. *Bon Appétit!*

Discharge Care Plan

For fun, please use your prioritizing nursing skill to reinforce some of the key messages of the chapter. Place what you think would be the correct prioritized number 1-5 in order of importance next to the corresponding letter.

A. __ Buy three or more healthy foods you have never tried before every time you go shopping.

B. __ Create a Code Brown "contamination" bin in your kitchen by getting rid of unhealthy foods.

C. __ Keep your blood sugar level by eating whole natural foods and reduce your added sugar intake.

D. __ Identify your unhealthy comfort foods and emotional comfort food triggers.

E. __ My emotional trigger is whenever I see blood. Maybe I should think of transferring out of the surgical unit!

Congratulations! You have earned a Golden Nightingale Wellness Wing by completing the interactive portions of the chapter!

(A = 1; B = 3; C = 4; D = 2; E = 5)

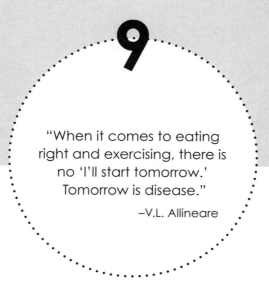

9

"When it comes to eating right and exercising, there is no 'I'll start tomorrow.' Tomorrow is disease."

–V.L. Allineare

Nourish Yourself, Nurse: Nutrition That Fits Your Life

The word *nursing* is derived from the Latin word *nutrire*, which means "to nourish." As a nurse, eating healthy can be extremely challenging, but you need to nourish yourself to have the energy and health to live well.

Nutrition 101

Here is a quick review of the macronutrients in basic nutrition:

- **Saturated fats:** Primarily found in animal sources, including red meat and whole dairy products. Saturated fats can raise your LDL cholesterol, which increases your risk of heart disease.

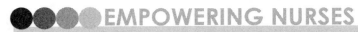

EMPOWERING NURSES

Dear Diary

Here are some food diary examples from nurses who have made healthy eating a part of their daily lifestyle.

Breakfast: Fresh fruit, oatmeal, and a protein mix made with light soy milk

Lunch: Healthy sandwich made on seven-grain bread, and low sodium tomato juice

Dinner: Lean filet mignon, fresh salad, green vegetable, and sweet potato

Breakfast: Egg white omelet with fresh asparagus, one piece whole grain bread, and fruit

Lunch: Organic eggs, egg salad with light mayonnaise, and whole grain toast

Dinner: Grilled red snapper, fresh greens, and brown rice

Dessert: Fresh strawberries with light whipped cream

"I have been able to integrate healthier fruits and vegetables. I try to bring my own food to work now. Our cafeteria is not conducive to a healthy meal. If I do eat there, I eat from the salad bar."

–Renee, resource nurse

Breakfast: Protein shake with berries or bananas or peanut butter

Lunch: Chicken with side of green beans, small side salad, and sugar-free Jell-O

Snack: Fruit

Dinner: Turkey tacos with wheat tortillas and beans

Dessert: Fruit or occasionally sugar-free fudgsical

"It's important not to starve yourself. I try to incorporate protein in every meal. It helps me feel full longer. I also try to eat small meals every few hours to keep my insulin from dropping and then snacking on whatever is lying around at work. It is important to pack your own lunch everyday and bring snacks. I also prepare meals ahead of time. I cook a bunch of fish, chicken, and turkey for the week. I also drink a lot of flavored water every day."

–Allison, clinical nurse manager, radiology

- **Trans fat:** Primarily found in packaged bake goods, commercially fried foods, processed foods, sweets, and so on. Made with partially hydrogenated vegetable oils. Trans fats can raise your LDL (bad) cholesterol and lower your HDL (good) cholesterol.

- **Monounsaturated fats:** Primarily found in olive oil, avocados, almonds, and pumpkin and sesame seeds. These fats can help lower the risk of heart disease.

- **Polyunsaturated fats:** Omega 3 and Omega 6 fatty acids. Found in cold water fish and fish oils, walnuts, and so on. These fats can help reduce risk of heart disease.

- **Refined carbs:** Stripped of bran, fiber, and nutrients. Found in foods made with white flour and white sugar. Refined carbs digest quickly and create an unhealthy roller coaster with your blood sugar levels, leading to possible weight gain, diabetes, and hypoglycemia.

- **Complex carbs:** A more natural state of foods—vegetables, fruit, whole grains, beans, and so on. Complex carbs digest slowly, making you feel full longer, and keep your blood sugar more level.

- **Dietary fiber:** Soluble (dissolves in water) or insoluble (cannot dissolve in water). Fiber can make you feel full faster which helps reduce caloric intake. Fiber also helps the passage of foods through the digestive system. Examples of soluble fiber are legumes, broccoli, artichokes, oats, rye, sweet potatoes. Examples of insoluble fiber are flaxseed, nuts, seeds, potato skins.

LIVEWELL

The *American Journal of Clinical Nutrition* reported a study by Sujatha Rajaram, Ella Haddad, Alfredo Mejia, and Joan Sabate (2009), which noted that including walnuts and fatty fish in a healthy diet lowered serum cholesterol and triglyceride concentrations, respectively, which affects heart disease risk favorably.

> **Trans Fats**
>
> According to the Nurses' Health Study Annual Newsletter 2007, trans fats can raise the level of LDL cholesterol and lower the level of HDL cholesterol. They can also cause inflammation to the cells that line the inner surface of the blood vessels, arteries, and veins. Nurses who consumed the most trans fats were 50% more likely to develop heart disease and 30% more likely to develop Type 2 diabetes than nurses who consumed the least trans fats.

Portion Control "Energy Plate"

Healthy portion size and eating high-performance foods is extremely important when it comes to your overall health and weight management. If you're not keeping track, it's very easy to eat more than you think. It's like spending on your credit card. You sometimes don't realize how much you have spent until you get the bill. In the case of food portion size, the bill you receive can be measured in pounds of extra body fat.

"The goal to healthy portion eating is to stop at the height of enjoyment."

To make healthy eating more simplified, buy a 10-inch divided plate. You can buy them at many general, grocery, or online stores, either reusable or disposable. The typical plate you use at home or at a restaurant is 12 or 14 inches. The portion control divided "Energy Plate" is a simple concept.

Figure 9.1

The divided Energy Plate.

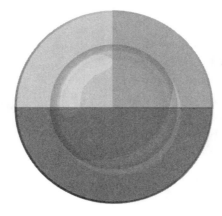

The Energy Plate allows for 400–500 calories per meal without having to count. The Energy Plate is divided into three sections:

- ¼ **healthy protein:** Lean meats, baked, broiled and grilled fish, tofu, egg whites, legumes, and so on.

- ¼ **whole grains:** Brown rice, whole grain bread, sweet potato, whole wheat pasta, and so on.

- ½ **vegetables and fruits.**

If you are still hungry after eating all the portions of the Energy Plate, add another helping of vegetables or fruit. If you cannot get your proteins, whole grains, vegetables or fruit in one meal, then you can make up for it at the next meal. Drinks count, too, so make your drinks healthy—water, flavored seltzer water, or noncaffeinated tea, and so on.

As a good reminder of eating healthy with the Energy Plate, place a divided paper plate on your refrigerator so every time you go to the refrigerator you are reminded of proper portion control and high-performance foods.

Teachers are taught to stop an activity at its height because it makes the children want to do the activity again. Otherwise, the activity could drag on and the children become less enthusiastic. I believe that holds true for portion control as well. You can eat past the point of feeling good, and then you are stuffed and feel sluggish and guilty that you ate too much. The goal to healthy portion eating is to stop at the height of enjoyment.

Portion control is really just healthy boundary setting. If you can be more assertive with implementing healthy boundary setting with people, the same can be true with boundary setting for healthier portion size.

Nutrition IV Bag

I've created a quick reference guide using an IV bag to inject Code Emerald foods instead of Code Blue foods. Code Emerald foods are energizing healthier gems of foods. Code Blue foods are unhealthy foods.

Figure 9.2

Try to imagine Code Blue foods flowing directly into the garbage bin, where they belong, and Code Emerald foods flowing directly into the blood stream for health and wellness.

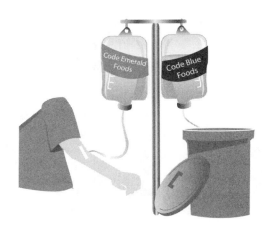

Code Blue foods:

- Regular and diet soda. Diet sodas do contain fewer calories than regular sodas. The problem with diet sodas is that they usually contain the artificial sweetener aspartame which is almost 200 times sweeter than sugar. This can help develop cravings for other sweet foods and unhealthy snacks which means consuming more calories

- Coffee

- Alcohol

- High-sugar or added sugar processed foods: sweets, ice cream, white breads, chips, and so on

- High-sugar cereals

- Highly saturated fatty meats: hot dogs, salami, sausage, bacon, and so on

- Fast food restaurants

- Fried foods

Code Emerald foods:

- Wild-caught cold water fish: wild salmon, cod, halibut, haddock, and so on

- Lean meats: no skin chicken, turkey, and so on

- Skinless game meats: duck, buffalo, venison, and so on

- Whole grains: brown rice, whole grain bread, whole wheat pasta, and so on

- Veggies and fruit

- Almonds and walnuts

- Hummus, avocados, almond butter

- Flaxseed

The Perils of the Hospital Cafeteria

Some hospital cafeterias are making an effort to serve healthier options for nurses and staff (Health Care Without Harm, www.noharm.org, has excellent resources for hospitals attempting to convert to healthier foods in their cafeterias). Unfortunately, though, some hospital cafeterias, despite the name changes, themed approaches, and even self-serve options, can still make you pretty sick.

Here is a quick tour of a hospital cafeteria I visited the other day:

- **Hours of operation:** First thing I noticed was the hours of operation: the cafeteria was open from 7:00 a.m.–6:30 p.m.—not the best fit for night shift nurses, even if they were tempted to eat there.

- **Sugar:** At the first stop, there's a choice of six different high-sugar, caffeinated soft drinks conveniently poured from a machine. (I don't know why they call them soft drinks because they're extremely hard on your system.)

- **Caffeine:** Next to the soft drinks are the caffeinated coffee drinks including three types of brewed coffee (one decaf). Caffeine may be your drug of choice but it picks you up, then slams you down—not to mention the negative impact it can have on your sleep patterns.

> "Caffeine may be your drug of choice, but it picks you up, then slams you down—not to mention the negative impact it can have on your sleep patterns."

- **Breakfast choices:** The breakfast food choices weren't much better. Ten high-sugar cereals, the average of them all containing a whopping 19 grams of sugar. The healthy option, a popular whole grain, organic cereal only had 6 grams of sugar per serving. Of course, there was also a choice of assorted sweet rolls, donuts, and white bagels, followed by juices that contain 34 grams of sugar per serving. The yogurts available had 25 grams of sugar per serving.

- **Desserts:** Then you go to the desserts: rice cereal treats, pies, cakes, and yogurt parfaits all loaded with sugar.

- **Grill:** Next were meal choices at the grill: Diners had a choice of artery thickening hot dogs, Polish sausage, French fries, cheese fries, and all topped off with the delicious but calorie laden, saturated fat king of the sandwiches: the Reuben! (They did have a vegetarian burger option as well.)

- **Pizza:** Next stop was the cheese and sausage laden pizza and choices of different types of chips with 220 milligrams of sodium per serving waiting for you.

- **Salad bar:** The salad bar seems like a saving grace until you realize that the choice of dressings are thousand island, caesar, blue cheese, and ranch. Pour a load of dressing on your salad, and you do yourself in. Where's the balsamic vinegar when you need it?

- **Fruit and finale:** You breathe a sigh of relief when you spot a lonely cup full of fruit. Unfortunately for the nurse who is hungry and whose blood sugar might be low from skipping a snack or a meal, that last stop—the "impulse buy" space right before the register is a freezer full of ice cream. (Time yourself; the longer you stand in line, the less likely you are to resist that temptation. Why aren't there bowls of fresh veggies in the impulse zone?)

I know I'm a little tough on the average hospital cafeteria. But all I want is two things for nurses. The first is to designate a section in the cafeteria for healthier options, and the second is to open the cafeteria for night shift nurses from 1:00 a.m.–3:30 a.m. Is this asking too much? I don't think so!

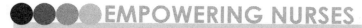

EMPOWERING NURSES

Ask and Ye Shall Receive!

Your cafeteria (or any institution) definitely won't change if you don't ask it to change. Kick in your assertive nurse training and ask for what you need. Start off with the cafeteria manager, asking for healthier low-sugar, low-fat foods (with more healthfully prepared vegetable options) and hours of operation for the night shift nurses. If that goes nowhere, don't give up. Instead, up the ante. Consider a petition asking for improved foods and hours of operation—get as many employees as possible to sign it. Consider asking your nurse managers to take up the cause on behalf of the staff. An organization called Health Care Without Harm (HCWH) has made significant strides in health care based activism and in designing tools for health care organizations to change their food policies in favor of more healthful options (http://www.noharm.org/). You may find some inspiration and useful tools at this Web site.

Fighting Depression

For those of you who have experienced depression and the devastating toll it takes on you, your work, and your loved ones, a healthier diet and regular exercise might help to improve mild depression.

Some foods can create extreme mood swings, especially refined carbs and sugars, including soft drinks, because of the roller coaster blood sugar levels that can aggravate symptoms of mild depression. Healthier foods can help improve your mild depression.

WebMD's Depression Guide (2009) includes articles on diet and depression (http://www.webmd.com/depression/guide/diet-recovery) and exercise and depression (http://www.webmd.com/depression/guide/exercise-depression), both are good resources. As we're focusing on nutrition in this chapter, here are a few key points to keep in mind about diet and depression management.

1. Stick to foods with high nutritional value, including foods high in minerals (including selenium), vitamins (especially vitamin D), Omega 3 fatty acids, and good quality proteins (legumes, turkey, chicken, tuna, and so on).

2. Eat "smart" carbs—whole grains, fruits, vegetables, and legumes—as they help boost serotonin levels in the brain.

3. The brain is particularly vulnerable to free radical damage. Eat foods rich in antioxidants (vitamins C, E, and beta carotene) to help support the brain, including:

   Beta carotene: apricots, broccoli, cantaloupe, carrots, collards, peaches, pumpkin, spinach, sweet potato.

   Vitamin C: blueberries, broccoli, grapefruit, kiwi, oranges, peppers, potatoes, strawberries, tomato.

   Vitamin E: nuts and seeds, vegetable oils, wheat germ.

4. Maintain a healthy weight and keep active to avoid the vicious cycle of obesity and depression.

Creating Your Nutrition Care Plan

Unlike all the diet books out there that promote their specific plan to lose 10 pounds in 10 seconds (ok, a slight exaggeration) or to eat 6 servings of dark chocolate throughout the day to drop your cholesterol 50 points, I believe no one-size-fits-all healthy nutrition plan exists. Every nurse has his or her own set of specific taste buds, lifestyle, and culture that come into play. In addition, everyone's body responds to different types of foods differently. However, I do firmly believe that the closer your food choice is to its natural state, the healthier you are going to be and the more energy you are going to possess.

With this thought process in mind, Raina Childers, RD, Director of Health Point Fitness, Southeast Missouri Hospital, and I have created a 7-day food variety menu for nurses who work during the day to serve as an example of one way of eating healthier. It does not take into account if you have specific food allergies, health issues, or weight goals. For example, I do not eat dairy or meat, so I would eliminate those from my menu. This is a general menu with specific measurements to give you a better idea of healthier portion sizes.

The daytime menu incorporates the "Energy Plate", which contains portion-sized protein, whole grains, fruits, or vegetables at every main meal.

Prep for the Week

One of the keys to eating healthier for nurses is to plan your meals every week so you don't grab unhealthy foods and snacks at work. The menu is based on 1,600–1,800 calories per day. Individual calorie needs are based on height, weight, age, and physical activity level. If possible, consult a nutrition expert to help you identify your specific needs.

LIVEWELL

Enhance Your Own Water

Use filtered water whenever possible. Remember that the bottled water may be nothing more than city water from some far-away place. To save the money and waste, buy yourself a sturdy reusable water bottle and pack your own water. If you want flavor, squirt in some fresh lemon or lime juice or drop in a noncaffeinated herbal tea bag or two in the morning when you fill your bottle. No need to brew the tea first. Just drop it in the water and the flavor will increase as the day goes on. Some of my favorites are peach, ginger, and raspberry herbal teas in water.

Water, flavored seltzer water, vitamin-fortified water, or noncaffeinated teas are all healthier options than the artificial energy boost and crash that soft drinks and caffeinated coffee offer. If you are drinking soft drinks, water might taste extremely bland to you. After you stop drinking soft drinks, you will find that water doesn't taste so bland.

LIVEWELL

Weighing Your Options

Kitchen scales can be useful in measuring portion size. There are many different scales based on how much money you want to spend and what style you prefer. Digital kitchen scales tend to be more precise than the mechanical models. You will measure food portions by their uncooked weight before you grill, bake, steam, or use your stove top.

MENU

Day 1

Breakfast: Two scrambled or omelet-style egg whites with veggies, one piece of whole grain bread with 1 tablespoon of reduced fat margarine (be sure it doesn't contain trans fats).

Snack: One apple and 2 tablespoons almond butter.

Lunch: One cup of low sodium vegetable soup, 2 cups mixed green salad with sliced tomato, cucumber, and 3 ounces of grilled chicken topped with ¾ tablespoons of light dressing.

Snack: Eight rice crackers (wafer sized crackers) and ½ cup of avocado dip.

Dinner: Four ounces baked/grilled fish with one cup steamed vegetables and 1 cup cooked brown or basmati rice, with ½ cup mushrooms and onions mixed in. One cup of fresh pineapple.

Day 2

Breakfast: One whole grain frozen waffle with strawberries on top or 2 tablespoons of reduced calorie syrup. Six ounces sugar- and fat-free yogurt with fresh fruit mixed in.

Snack: Fourteen raw almonds and 1 cup of low sodium tomato or V8 juice.

Lunch: Two slices whole grain bread with 1 tablespoon light or organic mayonnaise, 3 ounces of turkey breast with lettuce and tomato, and 1 cup of grapes.

Snack: Six figs.

Dinner: Six ounces of sautéed scallops, ½ cup long grain wild rice, 1 cup steamed asparagus, and 1 small whole grain roll with 1 tablespoon reduced fat margarine.

Day 3

Breakfast: One banana, ½ cup of whole grain cereal that has 6 grams of sugar per serving or less, 1 cup of fat-free milk, soy milk, or organic fat-free milk with no antibiotics or hormones.

Snack: ½ cup shelled edamame and 1 ounce of low-fat natural cheese.

Lunch: One whole wheat pita stuffed with tuna packed in water. Mix with 1 tablespoon light or organic mayonnaise and add tomato slices. ½ cup unsweetened applesauce.

Snack: Handful of sunflower seeds.

Dinner: Three ounces grilled chicken, 1 cup sautéed peppers and onions, 2 fajita-size whole wheat tortillas and ¼ cup salsa. One cup cucumber and tomato salad with balsamic vinegar.

Day 4

Breakfast: One cup steel cut oatmeal with 1 tablespoon chopped nuts and 1/2 cup fresh blueberries.

Snack: One cup baby carrots and ½ cup of hummus.

Lunch: Two cups romaine lettuce, ½ cup black beans, ½ tomato, 3 tablespoons light dressing, and 2 small, peeled kiwis.

Snack: Mix of eight almonds and eight walnuts.

Dinner: Four-ounce lean beef tenderloin, one 5-ounce baked, plain sweet potato. ½ cup steamed yellow squash. One cup fresh mixed berries.

Day 5

Breakfast: Two pieces of French toast made with whole grain bread and egg substitute, topped with fresh fruit or two tablespoons reduced calorie syrup. One 5-ounce peach/nectarine.

Snack: ½ plain sweet potato.

Lunch: One cup turkey chili (canned) and ½ almond butter and sugar-free jelly sandwich on whole grain bread. One cup grapes.

Snack: Sugar-free, fat-free yogurt and microwave frozen blueberries to mix in.

Dinner: Four ounces grilled chicken with two tablespoons BBQ sauce, ½ cup steamed corn, 1 cup steamed cauliflower, and 1 whole grain roll.

Day 6

Breakfast: One fruit smoothie with 1 teaspoon of wheat germ or ground up flaxseed and 1 piece whole grain toast.

Snack: ½ half cup Greek yogurt.

Lunch: Grilled chicken sandwich or wrap, lettuce, tomato, no mayonnaise. One apple, sliced.

Snack: Single serving package of microwave popcorn.

Dinner: Four ounces of baked/grilled wild salmon with one cup mixed steamed veggies and one cup brown rice. One sliced mango.

Day 7

Breakfast: Try a non-traditional breakfast to give you that extra boost in the morning. Homemade tuna salad mixed with veggies and light mayonnaise on one whole grain piece of bread and one cup of cubed cantaloupe.

Snack: Eight rice crackers and ½ cup salsa.

Lunch: Avocado sandwich made with ½ avocado, ¼ cup sauerkraut, mustard, or lettuce, tomato on two slices of whole grain bread.

Snack: Treat yourself as long as it doesn't trigger you to gorge, because sugar triggers you to eat more sugar—one low calorie, fat-free chocolate fudge bar.

Dinner: One veggie burger with lettuce and tomato on two slices of whole grain bread or bun. Small salad, one cup of brown rice, and a plum.

Eating vegan: Eating a vegan diet can be very challenging. There are a number of vegan cookbooks and lifestyle books. One of my favorite is *The Kind Diet* by Alicia Silverstone.

Restaurant Tips

The following tips were excerpted from the American Heart Association's (AHA) "Tips for Eating Out." AHA's site is very thorough and includes tips for eating out at various types of restaurants (http://www.americanheart.org/presenter.jhtml?identifier=531).

- Fried, au gratin, crispy, escalloped, pan-fried, sautéed or stuffed foods are high in fat and calories. Instead, look for steamed, broiled, baked, grilled, poached, or roasted foods. If you're not sure about a certain dish, ask your server how it's prepared. You can request that visible fat be trimmed from meat and skin be removed from poultry before cooking.

- Request that your meal be prepared with vegetable oil (made from canola, olive, corn, soy, sunflower, or safflower) or soft margarine instead of butter. Ask for soft margarine for your bread.

- High-sodium foods include those that are pickled, in cocktail sauce, smoked, in broth or au jus or in soy or teriyaki sauce. Limit these items. Ask that your food be prepared without added salt or MSG.

- Have gravy, sauces, and dressings served on the side, so you can control the amount you eat or skip them completely.

- Ask if the restaurant has fat-free or 1 percent milk instead of whole milk.

- Even if they aren't on the dessert menu, many restaurants can offer you fruit or sherbet instead of high-fat pastries and ice creams.

- Many supermarkets and specialty stores offer prepared entrees to take home when you're in a rush; the same tips listed here for restaurants also apply to take-home foods.

Non-Professional Resource

Throughout this book we offer you expertise on how to create a healthier lifestyle by health and wellness professionals. For nurses looking for a resource that gives you some nutritional tips from someone who has struggled with her weight and eating healthier you might want to check out Web sites and blogs from real people who are learning, struggling, and succeeding first hand! Lisa

Lillien's Hungry Girl Web site (www.hungrygirl.com) is one example, but there are 100s more out there. Lisa is not a nutritionist nor a doctor, and her Web site is not a substitute for professional guidance, but she provides her own experience and tips in an entertaining way.

It Loves Me, It Loves Me Not		
Trait	_Code Emerald_	_Code Blue_
Honesty	You can trust it to give you essential nutrients.	Cheats you of your essential nutrients.
Open Communication	Communicates with your blood sugar to keep it level.	Shuts down your ability to keep your blood sugar level, making you cranky and unhealthy.
Supportive	Helps raise your metabolism and lifts your moods.	Weighs you down with stored fats and always creates mood swings.
Financially Secure	Saves you money with your good health.	Runs up bills in medical costs, hospital stays, and prescription drug costs.
Good Energy	Gives you that extra spark.	Makes you feel run down and fatigued.
Nice Body	Looking fit.	Could use a body makeover.
Sensitive to Your Needs	It's healthy to go outside the relationship to get some of your emotional needs met.	Makes you co-dependent on food.
Family Values	Helps children to be healthy.	Doesn't like kids; ruins their health.
Humor	Laughter and eating healthy is good medicine.	No sense of humor makes you feel guilty.

Looking for Love in All the Wrong Places

We have such an abundance of unhealthy food choices that are instantly at our fingertips. Your grocery store likely has more than 50,000 food choices, many of them not always the healthiest for you. Unhealthy choices are sweet talking you to choose them when you fill up your tank, at the movies, nurses' stations, break rooms, patient rooms, vending machines, and hospital cafeterias. They are all whispering in your ear promises of fulfilling love that can tickle your taste buds if only you choose these bad boys. Because it's so easy for all of us to give into constant temptation, I'd like to feed you a fun and different spin on your relationship with food.

When you are in the process of choosing a relationship with a partner that you could spend the rest of your life with, your friends and family typically ask you to list the compatible characteristics you want and the non-compatible characteristics you don't want. With that in mind, I want you to think about your food as your love interest and check off the list of what you want in a life-long relationship with your food. Code Emerald implies a pattern of choosing healthier gems of high-performance energy dense foods, and Code Blue implies foods that are not the healthiest for you. Have fun!

Discharge Care Plan

For fun, to be formally discharged from this chapter please use your prioritizing nursing skill to reinforce some of the key messages of the chapter. Place what you think would be the correct prioritized number 1-4 in order of importance next to the corresponding letter.

A. __ Meal planning is essential for eating healthier because of your hectic schedule.

B. __ The 10-inch "Energy Plate" helps you with controlling portions and eating high-performance food: 1/4 protein, 1/4 whole grains, 1/2 veggies or fruits.

C. __ Eating whole natural foods enhances your health and boosts your energy.

D. __ The 42-inch plate is an effective portion-control tool for nurses who only have time to eat one meal a day because of a hectic schedule.

Congratulations! You have earned a Golden Nightingale Wellness Wing by completing the interactive portions of the chapter!

(A = 2; B = 1; C = 3; D = 4)

10

"Night-shift nurses deserve
their day in the sun!"

–Gary Scholar

When the Night Shift Eclipses You:
Special Strategies for Night-Shift Nurses

Like the mystical town in the musical *Brigadoon*, a world of
nurses exists at night while most of us are fast asleep. These are
nurses that are extremely busy giving night-time meds, changing IV solutions, handling unexpected admissions or emergen-
cies, comforting young patients, answering call lights, and handling a flood of other responsibilities. They are the *night-shift
nurses*. I devote this chapter to the night-shift nurses in the hope
of offering them a stronger voice to a group of hard working
and inspiring nurses who I believe are vastly underserved when
it comes to their own health and well-being.

> ### Sleep Deficits
>
> "When I worked the night shift, if I was not sleeping in preparation for the upcoming night shift, I was sleeping trying to catch up on my missed sleep. To make matters worse, if the assigned shifts were not on consecutive nights, or if I had any appointments, needed to run errands, or had any plans with family or friends, this feeling of exhaustion would set in like a thick fog. There was never enough time to feel 'normal.' Diet and fitness were never on my priority list; my energy was consumed in trying to catch up with my sleep."
>
> –Carmen, clinical and hospital nurse

According to Raina Childers, RD, nurses have found that some foods are harder for them to tolerate at night. So they start to decrease the variety of their diets. Many also use regular night feedings as a way to battle fatigue, eating more calories overall in a 24-hour period. They also complain of more gastroesophageal reflux disease (GERD) and gastrointestinal (GI) distress in general. Weight gain is a common issue for night-shift nurses. Caffeine abuse is prevalent, and can affect sleep patterns. Lack of sleep can then lower their resting metabolic rate and increase cravings for simple carbohydrates and fatty foods. It is a vicious cycle. The lack of healthy food choices on their shifts also comes into play. Many nurses eat out of vending machines and break rooms all night because the cafeteria is usually not open, and they don't have the energy or time to pack healthy snacks and lunches.

So what can you do if you're a night-shift nurse besides crawling into an empty bed on your shift and taking a much deserved nap or having your healthy food flown in from Canyon Ranch Spa? Because of all the challenges you face working your night shift, you need to be extremely diligent in your assertiveness for your own self care.

Assertive Nutritional Planning

I feel at my best when:

__ I try to take my meal breaks at the same time each night.

__ I do not skip meals because it keeps my blood sugar level, keeps my energy up, and helps me avoid excess hunger.

___ I avoid the notorious temptations of the vending machines of chips, soda, and sweets, or I request healthier options to be placed in the vending machines.

___ I drink plenty of water throughout my shift so I do not confuse dehydration for hunger.

___ I am assertive in my shopping and plan ahead to bring healthy foods from home.

___ I stop drinking caffeine altogether or I decrease caffeine as the shift progresses and stop drinking caffeine 4 hours before my shift ends so I can get a better night's sleep and not stay awake when I get home and eat unhealthy comfort foods.

___ I do not eat a large amount of food at the end of my shift. It can make it harder to sleep, and my body is less efficient at burning the calories during my less active times.

Mobile Munchies

Eating healthy can be frustrating because so many times those "scheduled" meal time breaks don't occur when they are suppose to because of the nature of nurse work. Sometimes you have a quiet night, and some nights all heck breaks loose and no one gets a break until after charting is completed and report is given to the incoming day-shift nurse.

For those times when sitting down for a 30-minute meal just doesn't work in your schedule, keep "mobile munchies" (healthy snacks) near your workstation. This way you won't experience intense physical hunger when your break does come, and you can make healthier choices. These mobile munchies are strictly a survival strategy you sometimes have to employ because of the nature of your work environment.

Combine whole grains/complex carbohydrates with lean proteins to provide sustained energy by keeping your blood sugar more level.

Mobile Munchies Suggestions

- Quaker Oatmeal squares dipped in 2 tablespoons of almond butter or natural (no sugar added) peanut butter.

- Whole grain (6-inch) tortilla with a 1/4 cup of fat-free refried beans.

- A serving of fruit with no sugar and no fat yogurt.

- No sugar, no fat yogurt with some raw nuts.

- Whole grain cereals (6 grams or less of sugar per serving) and 1/4 cup of raw nuts.

- Cut of veggies and fruit in an insulated container.

- Light soups in a can.

- Bag of raw (uncooked, unsalted) seeds and nuts.

Nutrition Care Plan

Raina Childers, RD, Director of Health Point Fitness, Southeast Missouri Hospital, and I have created a 7-day food variety menu for night-shift nurses to serve as an example of one way to eat healthier. This general menu has specific measurements to give you a better idea of healthier portion sizes. The night-shift menu incorporates the "Energy Plate" (refer back to Chapter 9 for a thorough discussion of the Energy Plate), which contains portion-sized protein, whole grain, and fruits or vegetables at every main meal.

Prep for the Week

One of the keys for night-shift nurses to eat healthier is to plan your meals every week. Pre-planning and packing of snacks and meals is required. However, some facilities have healthy meal choices offered during the night shift at a cafeteria or break area, and you might use that in lieu of bringing food for your meals. Another option—many night-shift workers find that frozen dinners work well for their meal breaks. If you are going to buy prepackaged frozen foods, do so carefully. Make sure you read the nutrition and ingredients lists thoroughly to be sure the sodium and sugars are appropriate for the serving level.

LIVEWELL

Weighing Your Options

Kitchen scales can be useful in measuring portion size. There are many different scales based on how much money you want to spend and what style you prefer. Digital kitchen scales tend to be more precise than the mechanical models. You will measure food portions by their uncooked weight before you grill, bake, steam, or use your stove top.

The night-shift menu is based on 1,600–1,800 calories per day. Individual calorie needs are based on height, weight, age, and physical activity level. If possible, consult a nutrition expert to help you identify your specific needs.

The night-shift menu is based on a 10:30 p.m. to 7:00 a.m. schedule. Adjust your own menu according to your shift. I encourage you to eat breakfast when you get home and then walk or perform low impact exercise, read, or relax for about one hour or more before going to sleep. Hopefully by following that pattern you will experience fewer interruption of your sleep.

Water, flavored seltzer water, vitamin-fortified water, or noncaffeinated teas are all healthier options than the artificial energy boost and crash that soft drinks and caffeinated coffee offer. If you are drinking soft drinks, water might taste extremely bland to you. After you stop drinking soft drinks, you will find that water doesn't taste so bland.

LIVEWELL

Enhance Your Own Water

Use filtered water whenever possible. Remember that the bottled water may be nothing more than city water from some far-away place. To save the money and waste, buy yourself a sturdy reusable water bottle and pack your own water. If you want flavor, squirt in some fresh lemon or lime juice or drop in a noncaffeinated herbal tea bag or two when you fill your bottle. No need to brew the tea first. Just drop it in the water and the flavor will increase as the day goes on. Some of my favorites are peach, ginger, and raspberry herbal teas in water.

NIGHT-SHIFT MENU

Day 1

Dinner (pre-work at home, as close to your shift start time as possible): Four ounces baked/grilled fish with 1 cup steamed vegetables and 1 cup cooked brown or basmati rice with ½ cup mushrooms and onions mixed in. One cup fresh pineapple.

Snack (12:00 a.m.): Eight rice crackers and ½ cup avocado dip.

Lunch (2:00 a.m.): One cup low sodium vegetable soup, 2 cups mixed green salad with sliced tomato, cucumber, 3 ounces of grilled chicken topped with 3 or 4 tablespoons of light dressing.

Snack (4:00 a.m.): One 5-ounce apple and 2 tablespoons almond butter.

Breakfast (home, 7:30 a.m.–8:30 a.m.): Two scrambled or omelet-style egg whites with veggies, 1 piece whole grain bread with 1 tablespoon of reduced fat margarine or low-sugar jam.

Day 2

Dinner (pre-work at home, as close to your shift start time as possible): Six ounces of sautéed scallops, ½ cup long grain wild rice, 1 cup steamed asparagus and. 1 small whole grain roll with 1 tablespoon reduced fat margarine.

Snack (12:00 a.m.): Six figs.

Lunch (2:00 a.m.): Two slices whole grain bread with one tablespoon light or organic mayonnaise, three ounces turkey breast with lettuce and tomato, one cup of grapes.

Snack (4:00 a.m.): Fourteen almonds and 1 cup low sodium tomato or V8 juice.

Breakfast (home, 7:30 a.m.–8:30 a.m.): One whole grain frozen waffle with strawberries on top or 2 tablespoons of reduced calorie syrup. Six ounces sugar- and fat-free yogurt with fresh fruit mixed in.

Day 3

Dinner (pre-work at home, as close to your shift start time as possible): Three ounces grilled chicken, 1 cup sautéed peppers and onions, 2 fajita-size whole wheat tortillas and ¼ cup salsa, 1 cup cucumber, and tomato salad with raspberry balsamic vinegar.

Snack (12:00 a.m.): Handful of sunflower seeds.

Lunch (2:00 a.m.): One whole wheat pita stuffed with tuna packed in water. Mix with 1 tablespoon light or organic mayonnaise and add tomato slices. ½ cup unsweetened applesauce.

Snack (4:00 a.m.): ½ cup shelled edamame and 1 ounce low-fat natural cheese.

Breakfast (home, 7:30 a.m.–8:30 a.m.): One 6-ounce banana, ½ cup whole grain cereal that has 6 grams of sugar per serving or less. One cup of fat-free cow (organic or without antibiotics and growth hormones), soy, or rice milk.

Day 4

Dinner (pre-work at home, as close to your shift start time as possible): Four-ounce lean beef tenderloin, one 5-ounce baked plain sweet potato. ½ cup steamed yellow squash, 1 cup fresh mixed berries.

Snack (12:00 a.m.): Mix of eight raw almonds and eight walnuts.

Lunch (2:00 a.m.): Two cups romaine lettuce, ½ cup black beans, ½ tomato, 3 tablespoons light dressing, 2 small peeled kiwi.

Snack (4:00 a.m.): One cup baby carrots and ½ cup of hummus.

Breakfast (home, 7:30 a.m.–8:30 a.m.): One cup steel cut oatmeal with 1 tablespoon chopped nuts and ½ cup fresh blueberries.

Day 5

Dinner (pre-work at home, as close to your shift start time as possible): Four ounces grilled chicken with 2 tablespoons BBQ sauce, ½ cup steamed corn, 1 cup steamed cauliflower.

Snack (12:00 a.m.): Sugar- and fat-free yogurt and microwave frozen blueberries to mix in.

Lunch (2:00 a.m.): One cup turkey chili (canned) and ½ tablespoon almond butter and sugar-free jelly sandwich on whole grain bread. One cup grapes.

Snack (4:00 a.m.): ½ plain sweet potato (cook, with skin pierced, in microwave).

Breakfast (home, 7:30 a.m.–8:30 a.m.): Two pieces French toast with whole grain bread and egg substitute, topped with fresh fruit or 2 tablespoons reduced calorie syrup. One 5-ounce peach/nectarine.

Day 6

Dinner (pre-work at home, as close to your shift start time as possible): Four ounces of baked/grilled wild salmon with 1 cup mixed steamed veggies and 1 cup brown rice. One sliced mango.

Snack (12:00 a.m.): Single serving package of microwave popcorn.

Lunch (2:00 a.m.): Grilled chicken or turkey sandwich or wrap, lettuce, tomato, no mayonnaise. One apple, sliced.

Snack (4:00 a.m.): ½ cup Greek yogurt.

Breakfast (home, 7:30 a.m.–8:30 a.m.): One fruit smoothie with 1 teaspoon of wheat germ or ground up flaxseed. One piece of whole grain toast.

Day 7

Dinner (pre-work at home, as close to your shift start time as possible): One veggie burger with lettuce and tomato on two slices of whole grain bread or bun. Small salad. One cup of brown rice and a plum.

Snack (12:00 a.m.): Treat yourself as long as it doesn't trigger you to gorge, because sugar triggers you to eat more sugar—one low calorie, fat-free chocolate fudge bar.

Lunch (2:00 a.m.): Avocado sandwich made with ½ avocado, lettuce, and tomato on two slices of whole grain bread.

Snack (4:00 a.m.): Eight rice crackers and ½ cup salsa.

Breakfast (home, 7:30 a.m.–8:30 a.m.): Try a non-traditional breakfast. Homemade tuna salad mixed with veggies and light or organic mayonnaise on one whole grain piece of bread and 1 cup cubed cantaloupe.

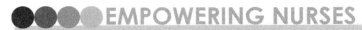

EMPOWERING NURSES

Eating Schedule for 12-Hour Shift: 7p.m.–7 a.m.

Dinner at home pre-work around 6:00 p.m.

Snack at midnight

Lunch between 2:00 a.m.–3:30 a.m.

Snack sometime before you head home.

Breakfast between 7:30 a.m.–8:30 a.m.

Alternative Eating Schedule for 12-Hour Shift

Breakfast in the afternoon when you wake up, between 3:30 p.m.–4:00 p.m.

Dinner at 9:00 p.m.

Lunch at 1:00 a.m.

Snack at 4:00 a.m.

This schedule leaves you 3–4 hours to digest your food before you go to sleep.

Sleep

Many nurses who work the night shift experience sleep deprivation because of the irregularity of their sleep hours and disruptions in their circadian rhythm.

Healthier foods and exercise work in tandem to provide you with better sleep:

- What you eat can affect your sleep patterns. Eating healthier, natural foods and keeping your blood sugar level by eliminating caffeine, alcohol, and high-sugar foods can help promote better sleep.

- You should avoid a heavy, high-fat meal before you sleep because it takes longer to digest and can affect your sleep. A heavy, high-fat meal needs to move more blood into your digestive tract and secrete more gastric acid and produce more digestive enzymes. The meal you eat before you go to bed should be light.

- Caffeine is an artificial stimulant that can keep you for getting a good night's sleep. Remember caffeine is found in coffee, some teas, and some chocolates.

- High-sugar foods or refined carbohydrates might disrupt sleep because your blood sugar level rises and then crashes, creating low blood sugar and causing you either to not get to sleep because of the high blood sugar level or to wake up in the middle of your sleep because of the low blood sugar level.

- Spicy foods can cause heartburn that keeps you from getting proper sleep.

- Foods that give you gas can keep you from proper sleep, for example, beans, eggplants, bananas, and some no-sugar desserts that use artificial sugars.

- Food allergies can also affect your sleep. Two common food allergies are dairy products and wheat.

- Exercise can promote better sleep because it raises your body temperature, which is followed by a drop in your body temperature a few hours later. When your temperature drops it signals your body to prepare for sleep.

- Exercise also eases muscle tension that can build up throughout your working shift. Easing muscle tension signals your body to prepare for sleep.

Lawrence Epstein and Steven Mardon explain in their acclaimed book, *The Harvard Medical School Guide to a Good Night's Sleep* (2007), "Sleep problems affect virtually every aspect of day to day living, such as mood, mental alertness, work performance, and energy level." Further, "Curtailing sleep to four hours a night for several nights results in changes in metabolism that are similar to those that occur in normal aging and that raise levels of hormones linked with overeating and weight gain. The overwhelming majority of individuals can get better sleep, if they're willing to make sleep a priority."

If you are experiencing sleep deprivation, I recommend the six-step plan for overcoming sleep issues in *The Harvard Medical School Guide to a Good Night's Sleep*.

> ### Sleeping
>
> "I am always feeling tired because of lack of sleep."
>
> —Steve, hospital RN, night shift
>
> "Night shift wreaks havoc on your sleep cycle."
>
> —Jamie, hospital RN, night shift

Creating a Night Shift Committee

Creating a Night Shift Committee at your hospital can play a vital role in advocating for the health and wellness of night-shift nurses. Here is an example of a Night Shift Committee created at AtlantiCare in New Jersey, contributed by Robyn Begley, DNP, RN CNEA-BC, vice president of nursing and CNO.

Creating the Night Shift Committee

- **2004:** Receive approval to design and implement a communication system capable of reaching night-shift staff during their working hours (without a budget).

- **2005:** The Night Shift Committee for Nursing Professionalism is formed with six members. Robyn approves electronic and voice signatures as validation of committee participation, which gives the freedom to make the new committee "night-shift friendly."

- **2006:** 22 members. Committee expands to multi-disciplinary.

- **2007:** 80 members. Present the program at the Magnet Conference.

- **2009:** 125+ members. The committee makes every effort to present information or opportunities for wellness during the night-shift nurses work hours.

Examples of Programs Available

- Health and wellness events
- Flu prevention fairs
- Unit specific education per request of a manager or a clinical specialist
- Informal surveys/pulse checks
- Access to committees
- Education on new products and equipment
- Nurse Week celebratory events
- Professional ladder projects

- Skills fairs

- Mandatory in-services

- Review and support during benefits enrollment

- Vendor access such as supplemental health and retirement planning

- Magnet, The Joint Commission, Stroke/Diabetic/One Call standards and initiatives

- Introduction of new or revised forms/policies/procedures

●●●●●EMPOWERING NURSES

"We asked our organization to support health and wellness events during night-shift hours. We now have B/P, cholesterol, and blood sugar screenings along with education of the risk factors associated with working the night shift. Our organization owns a life center gym, and they opened it for hours that are supportive of the night-shift staff. We also asked our organization to open the cafeteria up at night. The hours are 1 a.m. to 3 a.m. This gives us better choices and access to fresh fruit and salads."

–Cathy, RN, night-shift liaison

Discharge Care Plan

For fun, to be formally discharged from this chapter please use your prioritizing nursing skill to reinforce some of the key messages of the chapter. Place what you think would be the correct prioritized number 1-5 in order of importance next to the corresponding letter.

A. __ Plan your meals every night so you are not tempted by unhealthy foods at the vending machines, break room, or nurses station.

B. __ Bring a mobile munchy healthy snack to keep your blood sugar level and energy up. Combine whole grain/complex carbs and lean protein.

C. __ Stop drinking caffeinated sodas and coffee or reduce drinking caffeine beverages as your shift progresses. Do not eat a large amount of food toward the end of your shift.

D. __ Create a Night Shift Committee for the health and wellness of the night-shift nurses.

E. __ My new night-shift hours are 7 p.m.–8 p.m. Working only one hour a night gives me a better opportunity to eat healthier and allows me to watch my favorite TV shows, *E.R.* and *Scrubs*.

Congratulations! You have earned a Golden Nightingale Wellness Wing by completing the interactive portions of the chapter!

(A = 1; B = 2; C = 3; D = 4; E = 5)

11

"I honor myself when I honor
my own body image!"

–Gary Scholar

Weighing Your Options: Weight Management for Every Nurse

An overweight nurse I know wouldn't take responsibility for her unhealthy eating patterns. So I asked her, "Who does the grocery shopping in your family?"

She replied, "I do."

"Who brings the groceries into your house?"

She replied, "I do."

"Who cooks your meals?"

She replied, "I do."

"And who puts the food into your mouth?"

She replied, "I do."

"Then whose responsibility is it that you're eating unhealthy?"

She replied, "It's my husband's fault because he drives me crazy!"

While this story may be funny, it clearly makes the point that we all have to take responsibility for our own actions, including putting our bodies in the best possible position to succeed in weight management. Knowledge is power, so this chapter examines healthy weight management.

Planning and Control

If you plan to lose body fat percentage, you need to first give yourself a firm date to start. With weight-loss management, planning and prepping meals for the week is extremely important because it helps you stay on track. Losing weight is a slow process if you are doing it in a healthy way—a rate of 1–2 pounds a week is optimal. So to be on top of your weight management and feel in control, you need to stay focused on your goal of being healthier every day. It is certainly easy for outside distractions and people to sabotage your efforts, inadvertent or not.

Use your assertive skills to be accountable to keep on track of your weight loss and weight management progress.

Exercise and Reward

Are you one of those nurses who is exercising but not losing body fat percentage? If you work out and then reward yourself and eat a large amount of calories at a fast food restaurant or finish off a pint of ice cream, that negates some of the benefits you achieved when working out. Even if you're eating healthier, overindulging is counterproductive to losing body fat. Remember food and portion size count. Also, you might have reached a plateau with the intensity and duration of your workout and need to change the activity or increase intensity and duration.

●●●●●EMPOWERING NURSES

Assertive Accountability Weight Loss Progress

Motivation Goal: (specific health measure, energy, clothes size, and so on)

_____

Fit by: (assertive yet realistic time frame: by age 40, before class reunion, before child's college graduation and/or wedding, and so on)

_____

Start Date: _____

Goal Date (specific date or general time period): _____

Weight Loss Goal: _____

Body Fat % Goal: _____

Weight Management Progress: _____

Starving Yourself Is Not the Answer

If you are starving yourself (eating below 1,200 calories a day), the result is not going to be the weight loss you desire because your body has learned to conserve itself by not burning fat. You are only teaching your body to hold on to your unwanted pounds. Your body has no idea when it is going to eat again, so it thinks, "Hey, I have to survive so I'm going to adapt and lower the metabolism and store fat, which gives me a fighting chance to survive this crazy diet!" Diets that are extremely restrictive also create temptation to overindulge because you feel deprived both emotionally and physically. For your own sake, please take a new approach and eat small healthy meals throughout the day that total more than 1,200 calories, which boosts your metabolism.

Program Yourself for Long-Term Success

Identifying what made you gain weight in the first place is ultimately what will help you keep off your weight when you have lost it. The last thing you want to happen after working so hard to lose your weight is to disappoint yourself by gaining the weight back and more. Then the guilt and beating yourself up is looped over and over again in your mind. Those who have been successful in long-term weight management understand that maintaining your healthier weight takes as much work and vigilance as losing the weight. For example, if you are using a food diary for weight loss it can be just as important to use it while maintaining your healthier weight.

6 Keys to Successful Long-Term Weight Management

1. Remember that assertiveness is just as important to weight maintenance as it is to losing weight. Assertiveness gives you a heightened sense of feeling in "control," which is vital when it comes to long-term weight management success. Assertiveness takes you to the next level by conveying your inner feelings, beliefs, and goals to yourself and others in a positive, clear, and direct way. It will allow you to continue getting your needs met during your weight management phase by taking ownership of your daily choices.

2. Establish a healthy balanced diet that you enjoy. Remember to always buy 3 or more healthy foods you have never tried before each time you go shopping. This way you will choose those healthier foods you really enjoy and won't have the tendency to get bored with your choices. Besides, it makes grocery shopping so much more interesting and fun!

3. Do not make exercise drudgery. Schedule regular exercise you enjoy. Without the enjoyment, you will end up sabotaging your efforts by finding excuses not to exercise.

4. Eat a healthy breakfast every day. It boosts your mood and metabolism and sets you up for the remainder of your day and night.

5. Create a healthy support system that welcomes the encouragement of family, friends, and co-workers.

6. Self monitor your emotional situations and feelings that trigger you to overeat when you are physically not hungry. This is the one key to long-term successful weight management that usually is the most difficult to be consistent with because it is usually one of the most powerful reasons people overeat in the first place. Nurses may use food to help cope with the fears, insecurities, and stress in their lives. When you hold onto your fears, insecurities, and stress, the tendency is also

to hold onto your pounds. Creating new habits or making paradigm shifts on how you cope with, let go of, or forgive your fears, insecurities, and stress can help you grow and transform your life, happiness, and health. While your job is to help save and improve patients' lives, it's also your responsibility to care for that part of yourself you may have left behind—your emotional self!

Career Impact on Weight Management

Throughout this book, you have read stories in which nurses discuss the impact of nursing on their emotional and physical health. Each and every nurse whose voice is represented in this book had to make implementing self-care a priority. This is especially true when it comes to weight. Many nurses can blame their weight gain on their jobs. They may overeat in an attempt to compensate for stress, long hours, or unhappiness. Or they may have a difficult time losing that weight because they are in the habit of turning to food for comfort.

That's why it is imperative that you are assertive in meeting your needs when it comes to your own career. For example, one way to reduce your stress might be through creating more open communication with your charge nurse or nurse administrators. Schedule a meeting with them to develop a plan for using more of your strengths as a nurse. Or, you may be in a situation where you're not happy; in that case, you may want to explore the possibilities of applying for another shift or department. Perhaps your dream job is to be a school nurse—you will need to use your assertive skills to network, be persistent, and apply for those jobs as they become available. You may want to direct your energy toward attaining additional degrees or credentials to become a nurse executive. Developing wellness or wellness support programs is another option that might help meet both your needs and those of your co-workers. Or, you could transform a break room into a relaxing tranquility room—complete with meditative music, aromatherapy, and chair massages—where nurses can decompress from their hectic, stressful work during breaks.

The important message is that weight management is so much more effective for nurses whose career path fits their needs. You will find it much easier to manage your weight when you are happy in your life, including your career.

Your Subconscious Mind

Your mind and thoughts affect your eating habits and weight management as well. Ryan Roessler, a certified hypnotherapist and founder of Wellsprings Hypnosis in Chicago, Illinois, explains:

> Hypnosis is a way to get past your conscious mind, which judges and can be critical, to your subconscious mind, which is emotional and uncritical. To achieve healthier eating, regular fitness, and weight management you need both your conscious and subconscious mind working in tandem. By relaxing the conscious mind, we can give the subconscious mind what we call suggestions. The suggestions reinforce what you consciously want and convince the subconscious mind to go along with it. The suggestions after they have slipped past the conscious mind tend to change your behaviors of using food as a crutch or emotional eating by unlocking what you are blocking. The suggestions are combined with ego enhancement because a compliment or positive reinforcement given to your subconscious mind is 10 times more powerful than one given to the conscious mind. (personal communication, n.d.)

Nightingale Living Well Pledge

Losing weight and keeping it off are difficult goals to attain. You need to feel you have control over your success, so I believe any positive tools you can use in your weight management first-aid kit are going to benefit you.

Many graduating nurses still take the Nightingale Pledge. As a conscious and subconscious tool, I wrote the Nightingale Living Well Pledge. Please take a few minutes to recite this new pledge to yourself when you wake up and before you go to bed.

Karen, the nurse executive we met in Chapter 1, is a great example of a nurse effectively managing her weight. She has lost 40 pounds with a 6 point reduction in her Body Mass Index (BMI) and 13 inches in her body circumference. She has also decreased her LDL cholesterol. She accomplished it by reaching out for support and working with my colleague Raina Childers, RD, by learning how to be assertive for her own self care, eating healthier, and by scheduling in fitness. Karen is 66 years "young," yet she serves as a role model to those at any age, proving that you can implement a healthier Lifestyle Shift no matter how hectic your work schedule.

Nurses' Living Well Nightingale Pledge

I solemnly pledge to give myself this moment, a soft place to land each day so I can reflect and collect thoughts that will empower me forward.

I have the power of choice to retrain my taste buds by choosing delicious healthy comfort foods that provide me with energy, health, and vitality.

I will be assertive in the pursuit of healthy portion sizes and will eat only until I am comfortably satisfied. Then I will give myself the gift of healthy boundary setting by stopping eating, which sets me free from the guilt of overeating.

I will buy three or more new healthy foods I've never tried before every time I go shopping.

I will schedule physical activity I enjoy that will energize me, reshape my body, and raise my endorphins to help me feel better.

I will let go of all past experiences, negative thoughts, and excuses that limit my capacity to reach my potential of optimal health and well-being.

I will be especially gentle on myself when it comes to my own body image. Being fit isn't about trying to have the perfect body. It's about taking care of the body I have!

I will reach out and ask for support and encouragement in my journey of living well.

I will devote myself to the commitment of my own self care and getting my needs met because I truly deserve it.

I am all powerful by spreading my Nightingale wings and soaring to new heights of living well on the assertive winds of change!

–Gary Scholar

Listen To Your Body

You can place enormous stress on yourself to be near perfect in your job as a nurse. That internal pressure of perfectionism can transfer into your personal life in the form of constant looping. Consider your sabotaging self thoughts from waking up in the morning and finding your clothes don't fit, constantly

> ### Toothpaste Technique
>
> An effective way to stop eating after you have eaten healthy portion sizes is to immediately brush your teeth. The sudden change of the toothpaste to your taste buds signals you to stop eating.

weighing yourself, counting calories, and using comfort food to feel better when you're overwhelmed. Add to that the cultural messages that can make you feel your body is not good enough the way it is, and these messages can set you up for the roller coaster of yo-yo dieting, which teaches you to disregard both your emotional needs and making a healthy nutritional Lifestyle Shift. In addition, severe roller-coaster dieting and poor body image can lead to eating disorders.

A good idea when it comes to your own struggles with weight management is to listen to the red flags your own body is trying to tell you.

> Hello, it's me—your body talking! I know you don't really give me much thought, but I have feelings, too! So I want to seize this moment and have a heart-to-heart chat with you because I've got a few things I need to get off my chest. First off, I'm working for you 24/7, day and night shifts, with no time off. Talk about sleep deprivation! I'm constantly multitasking and prioritizing the care plan for all of your organs. If it's not your heart that needs constant attention, it's your blood pressure or cholesterol levels. If that's not enough, I'm always dealing with new emergency admissions of overdosing your blood sugar because of your unhealthy processed and junk food eating. And then you have the small matter of trying to manage your weight. You're constantly so hard on yourself, which has a negative effect on me. You loop about how your clothes aren't fitting properly, how you look compared to celebrities, or how you have a wedding or high school reunion coming up and you've got to look good.
>
> So then you force me go on one of those one-size-fits-all, raspberry yogurt starvation diets. And you end up blaming and giving me guilt when you stop dieting and gain all your weight back and then some. You know, calories-in and calories-out isn't the entire equation. Did you ever realize that healthy weight management is very individualized? What

works for cousin Sue or uncle Mark might not work for you. I mean, check your body chart. You've got food sensitivities to lactose/dairy. Your chronic stress at work is causing high levels of cortisol, you're not getting adequate sleep, and you've got hormonal imbalances affecting your metabolism because of lack of exercise and your unhealthy starvation dieting.

I know. Who am I to complain? I admit it! I'm an enabler. I try to fix anything you throw my way, and I give and give and give. But to be perfectly honest I've come to the end of my toes, and I feel completely overwhelmed and burnt out. That's why you've felt the heartburn, headaches, and fatigue lately. So for once in my life, I'm going to take care of myself and be assertive in asking you to meet my needs when it comes to your weight management. By the way, it's not about dieting—it's about working your Lifestyle Shift of eating healthier, exercising regularly, and placing self care higher on your priority list. Hey, don't forget I can read, too!

I'm glad we finally had this heart-to-heart chat. I always feel better when I can talk things out instead of keeping things bottled up inside. Let the list below, in "Assertiveness Training," be your list to yourself of your needs.

Assertiveness Training:

I feel at my best when:

_____ I change my focus from dieting to making permanent lifestyle changes of eating healthier that I can sustain for the rest of my life. These changes place my priority on health and energy, instead of my weight.

_____ I make a paradigm shift to put getting my needs met at the top of my priority list to curb my unhealthy comfort eating.

_____ I don't skip meals, and I make sure I eat more than 1,200 calories a day.

_____ I don't obsess about the scale. A better indicator of body fat loss is how my clothes fit.

_____ I make it a commitment to myself that I don't beat myself up over my body image. If my body changes as a result of working my Lifestyle Shift I leave that in the future. As of today, I accept what my body looks like now.

_____ I drink water or seltzer water instead of sodas, caffeinated coffee, and alcohol. Lack of water promotes fat deposits in my body.

_____ I keep my blood sugar levels even by eating high-fiber, low-sugar foods and focusing on appropriate portion-sized meals every 3–4 hours. If I don't, my blood sugar gets too low, making me want to binge as fast as I can to bring my blood sugar up.

_____ I use a 10-inch divided "Energy Plate" for portion control.

_____ I stop eating 2–3 hours before I go to bed; otherwise, I store the food as fat and end up not eating breakfast in the morning because I'm not hungry.

_____ I exercise to my target heart rate at least 30 minutes a day, and build up to 45 minutes to one hour a day. If you want to lose weight, fat burning needs that much time to kick in. I realize the strongest indicator of long-term weight management, health, and energy level is through physical activity.

_____ I am assertive and communicate to my family, friends, and co-workers that making changes can be a challenge and I need their support. I model working my Lifestyle Shift and invite them into the process.

_____ I keep a food diary. I can do this by writing down what I ate. This activity makes me more aware of what I eat and the portion sizes.

_____ I keep a "Photo Food Diary" by taking photos with my cell phone camera of the food and portion size I eat.

_____ I snack on a good book or hobby, listening to music, and so on instead of snacking on unhealthy food.

Coping with the Death of a Patient

One of the most stressful components of a nurse's job is coping with the death of a patient. It creates grief-related stress, and the stress can influence overeating.

In some cases you might be the last compassionate face that patients see before they pass away. You comfort patients in their last moments and have the heavy burden of comforting their loved ones afterwards. I'm not going to sugarcoat this because I've heard from too many nurses about the emotional toll it takes on them—no matter whether they are in their first week on the job or they have been a veteran for 30 years in the profession.

●●●●●EMPOWERING NURSES

Grieving

In my experience, the hospital setting is very hectic and there was never time to deal with the feelings of a patient's death. I was always moving on to the next patient, the next task, or whatever. I hope that is changing, and there is more support for nurses.

In hospice, where I work currently, there is much support for nurses after a patient's death. We do a lot of verbal processing with one another and have the support of the social workers on our team. We also talk a lot about boundaries and how not to get overly involved emotionally with our patients, though at times it's difficult to do.

Many times the nurses will attend the funeral for closure, or they may take an extra day off or need a lighter caseload after a patients' death. Every week, we hold a memorial service to remember those who have died. We honor that person, and if it was difficult, there is more sharing. I feel grateful to work in an environment where nurses can express their feelings and get support.

–Bonnie, RN hospice nurse

The Department of Nursing at Roswell Park Cancer Institute, Buffalo, New York, created a pilot program that provides emergency emotional support for nurses immediately after a patient's death. It's called the Code Gray Program and involves intervention and peer-based support immediately after death. Upon death of the patient, the Take Charge Nurse conducts an assessment of the emotional needs of the nurse. During a 20-minute break the nurse can talk to a support team or spend time off the floor. Then at the end of the shift, a reassessment is taken to determine the need for ongoing support.

Every nurse copes with patient deaths differently, but here are some suggestions for ways to support your own needs during this difficult time.

- Voice your feelings and get support from your co-workers.

- If needed, seek out professional help.

- Try to stay in touch with your own feelings of death and dying.

- If applicable to you, turn to your faith and prayer.

- Create programs for your staff or co-workers that involve grief preparation and training of nurses.

- Have senior nurses mentor younger nurses about the grieving process.

The Hospice Foundation of America (www.hospicefoundation.org) provides valuable links, articles, and resources for dealing with loss.

Nurses Coping with Their Own Eating Disorder

Throughout the years, I've witnessed the devastating toll that eating disorders can take on nurses' lives. Nurses who have an eating disorder struggle with hiding it because of shame and guilt, which promotes heartbreaking feelings of isolation, loneliness, hopelessness, and despair. Eating disorders can also have a negative ripple effect on nurses' families.

The emotionally and physically demanding, high-stress, crazy hours, life and death profession of nursing can add to the dysfunction of a nurse's eating disorder. Nurses who have an eating disorder might use it as a coping mechanism to help manage their stress and anxiety.

Raina Childers, RD explains:

> I often get referrals to cooperatively work with a psychologist or licensed therapist with their client who has an eating disorder. My goal, when working together with mental health professionals, is to work the 'binge,' the 'purge,' and the 'self-starvation' coping mechanism out of a 'job.' So many individuals who have an eating disorder begin to define themselves by the way they manage their stress and anxiety. When they think of giving up a familiar coping mechanism, they panic and feel they will lose control. Many of them can't immediately see how out of control they really are until they start their road to recovery (personal communication, n.d.).

If you are a nurse that has an eating disorder, I want you to take heart in the fact that many individuals have taken back their lives when faced with an eating disorder. I also want you to know you are not alone, and professional help can treat your eating disorder. Treatment for an eating disorder can be provided through psychological and nutritional counseling from health professionals, group therapy, outpatient therapy, or inpatient therapy. Here are some other resources you can seek out if you feel you need help:

- National Eating Disorders Association (NEDA) (www.NationalEatingDisorders.org), Information and Referral Helpline: 800-931-2237—The NEDA is a non-profit organization dedicated to supporting individuals and families affected by eating disorders.

- Overeaters Anonymous (OA) (www.oa.org)—OA offers a program of recovery from compulsive eating using the Twelve Steps and Twelve Traditions of Alcoholics Anonymous. OA offers approximately 6,500 meetings in over 75 countries that provide a fellowship of experience, strength, and hope where members respect one another's anonymity. OA is not just about weight loss, weight gain, obesity, or diet. It addresses physical, emotional, and spiritual well-being. Online or telephone meetings are also offered.

- The American Psychiatric Association (www.psych.org).

- The National Institute of Mental Health (www.nimh.nih.gov).

Definitions of Eating Disorders

The National Eating Disorder Association defines the following eating disorders:

- **Anorexia Nervosa** is a serious, potentially life-threatening eating disorder characterized by self-starvation and excessive weight loss.

- **Binge Eating Disorder (BED)** is a type of eating disorder not otherwise specified and is characterized by recurrent binge eating without the regular use of compensatory measures to counter the binge eating.

- **Bulimia Nervosa** is a serious, potentially life-threatening eating disorder characterized by a cycle of bingeing and compensatory behaviors such as self-induced vomiting designed to undo or compensate for the effects of binge eating (2009a).

Symptoms of an Eating Disorder

Bulimia

- Repeated episodes of binging and purging
- Feeling out of control during a binge and eating beyond the point of comfortable fullness
- Purging after a binge (typically by self-induced vomiting; abuse of laxatives, diet pills, and/or diuretics; excessive exercise; or fasting)
- Frequent dieting
- Extreme concern with body weight and shape

Anorexia

- Resistance to maintain body weight at or above minimally normal weight for height, body type, age, and activity level
- Intense fear of weight gain or being "fat"
- Feeling "fat" or overweight despite dramatic weight loss
- Loss of menstrual periods
- Extreme concern with body weight and shape

Binge Eating Disorder (BED) (also known as compulsive overeating)

- BED is characterized primarily by periods of uncontrolled, impulsive, or continuous eating beyond the point of feeling comfortable.

Though compulsive overeaters do not purge, they might engage in sporadic fasts or repetitive diets and often experience feelings of shame or self-hatred after a binge.

People who overeat compulsively might struggle with anxiety, depression, and loneliness, which can contribute to their unhealthy episodes of binge eating.

Body weight can vary from normal to moderate or severe obesity.

(National Eating Disorder Association, www.NationalEatingDisorders.org)

Contributing Causes of Eating Disorders
Psychological Factors
- Low self-esteem
- Feelings of inadequacy or lack of control in life
- Depression, anxiety, anger, or loneliness

Interpersonal Factors
- Troubled family and personal relationships
- Difficulty expressing emotions and feelings
- History of being teased or ridiculed based on size or weight
- History of physical or sexual abuse

Social Factors
- Cultural pressures that glorify "thinness" and place value on obtaining the "perfect body"
- Narrow definitions of beauty that include only women and men of specific body weights and shapes
- Cultural norms that value people on the basis of physical appearance and not inner qualities and strengths

Biological Factor
- Eating disorders often run in families. Research indicates significant genetic contributions to eating disorders.

(National Eating Disorder Association, www.NationalEatingDisorders.org)

Discharge Care Plan

For fun, to be formally discharged from this chapter please use your prioritizing nursing skill to reinforce some of the key messages of the chapter. Place what you think would be the correct prioritized number 1-6 in order of importance next to the corresponding letter.

A. __ Physical activity is one of the strongest indicators of long-term weight management.

B. __ Keeping my blood sugar level throughout the day helps with not overeating between or at meals.

C. __ I change my focus from dieting to making permanent lifestyle changes of healthier eating that I can sustain for the rest of my life.

D. __ I make a commitment not to beat up myself over my body image.

E. __ I will not starve myself to try to lose weight. I will eat smaller, more balanced meals throughout the day.

F. __ Losing unhealthy body fat can become quite expensive because now you'll be able to fit into that amazing dress or suit you always wanted to buy in the upscale department store!

Congratulations! You have earned a Golden Nightingale Wellness Wing by completing the interactive portions of the chapter!

(A = 2; B = 3; C = 1; D = 4; E = 5; F = 6)

12

"Nutritional balance gives you the inner compass to attain optimal health!"

–Gary Scholar

Holistic Health and Nutrition From Traditional Chinese Medicine

–Caroline Jung, LAc, MSOM Certified Acupuncturist, Masters of Science in Oriental Medicine

Traditional Chinese Medicine (TCM) practitioners look at the whole person when considering treatment. I was first attracted to TCM in high school. I was interested, particularly, in how TCM identified nutrition and food choices as an integral part to your overall health. Since then, I have learned a whole new way of looking at and choosing foods. Chinese nutrition is different from Western nutrition in a number of aspects, but two in particular.

LIVEWELL

TCM treats both the root and the branch of the problem from a holistic perspective.

1. TCM categorizes food by its properties, characteristics, flavors, and so on.

2. TCM takes into account each individual person's constitution—physical characteristics, spirit, mental state, and so on—which is really impacted by food choices.

A Holistic Approach to Nurses' Lifestyle and Health

When we treat patients from a Chinese medicine perspective, we do a thorough questioning and consultation. We look at your body from a holistic view whatever the treatment approach—whether we are using acupuncture, nutrition, or a combination of therapies. We treat the root and branch of any illness. For example, if you have a migraine headache, the root of the headache is what *is causing* the headache and the branch *is* the headache itself. With TCM, we treat your entire body system, which comprises your body, mind, and spirit. These three parts of you depend on one another, support one another, and nourish one another. All three aspects of every individual must be balanced to have optimal health. After you have one component balanced, it makes it that much easier to balance the other aspects as well. If one part falls out of balance, it is easy for it to cause another part to fall out of balance, too. It is like a constant juggling act to keep the three parts harmonious, but by making healthy nutritional selections and lifestyle choices, you can keep the three parts of your system stable.

"Chinese nutrition blends into your lifestyle because it plays a part of how you feel, physically and emotionally, based on your food choices, and all of that plays a part regarding your general attitude and approach and how you set yourself up to feel for work and for personal priorities."

I look at Chinese nutrition as a part of your lifestyle. So, it is not only about the food you choose, but also about how you incorporate their functions and the meaning of their functions into your diet. Lifestyle is so important to how you feel each day. It is the foundation of your well-being. Your lifestyle can include very few or a great many aspects depending on how simple you want it to be. Lifestyle is a way of life or style of living that reflects the attitudes and values of a person or group. Chinese nutrition blends into your lifestyle because it plays a part of how you feel, physically and emotionally, based on your food choices, and all of that plays a part regarding your general attitude and approach and how you set yourself up to feel everyday for work and for personal priorities. TCM always takes into account your mind, body, and spirit connection.

LIVEWELL

Body, Mind, and Spirit

In TCM, all three aspects of each individual—body, mind, and spirit—must be balanced for optimal health to occur.

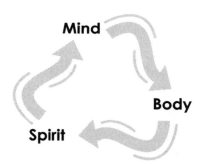

Figure 12.1

The smooth energy flow between the mind, body, and spirit. This illustrates how all three nourish and support one another.

Nutrition is a fundamental part of your health. It is the foundation upon which all of your physical, emotional, and spiritual energies rely for your daily functions, growth, and development. Chinese nutrition views your health and body from a holistic view. We look at the mind, body, and spirit. As noted earlier, these three parts of every individual are connected. If you have an excess and/or deficiency in any area of your body, it in turn causes an excess and/or deficiency in another part of your body. For example, if you are in an accident and break your ankle, you might become depressed because you can't physically do everything you are accustomed to doing. Or, if you develop anxiety, you might lose your appetite or just stop eating all together to cope with your anxious feelings. So the mind, body, and spirit connection is one harmonious circle of energy from one part feeding off the other ones.

Understanding Basic TCM Terminology and Concepts

Before going into detail about foods, I want to present some basic terminology we use in TCM. You might already be familiar with some of the terms. Chinese nutrition falls under the umbrella of TCM, which includes many modalities such as moxibustion and cupping. Both are forms of therapy we use in conjunction with acupuncture and herbs. The following are a few basic terms.

- *Qi*, pronounced chi, is a Chinese word that means life energy, also referred to as vital energy. This is the energy we talk about that runs through your channels and is what we are balancing when we use acupuncture to "balance your energy."

- *Channel*, *meridian*, and *vessel* all have the same meaning—they are the pathways that run throughout your body. These pathways carry your qi, and they are the courses (pathways) that have your acupuncture points on them. In acupuncture, we insert fine, thin needles into the points along your meridians to balance your qi.

- *Yin* and *yang* comprise a philosophical method to analyze and understand everything that happens in our natural world. Yin and yang are sometimes referred to as yin and yang energies, but technically, the "energy" in question has either yin and/or yang qualities to it. Yin and yang represent a way to understand the opposite ends of any phenomenon in our world. For example, yin is cold and is active at nighttime whereas yang is hot and active during the daytime. Yin and yang explain how things function in relation to each other and to the changes in nature. They are one another's support and supply of energy. They also have feminine and masculine qualities, yin being feminine and yang being masculine.

> "Yin and yang represent a way to understand the opposite ends of any phenomenon in our world. For example, yin is cold and is active at nighttime whereas yang is hot and active during the daytime. Yin and yang explain how things function in relation to each other and to the changes in nature."

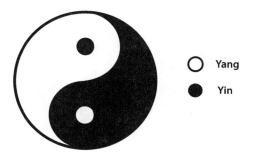

Figure 12.2

Yin and yang represent a way to understand the opposite ends of any phenomenon in our world.

Considering Food Properties, Characteristics, and Flavors

A Chinese nutritional approach looks at all properties, characteristics, and flavors of foods. This approach tends to differ from Western nutrition in that TCM pays attention to and looks at how the food reacts to every cell, organ, tissue, and energy in the body. To begin with, TCM looks at the hot and cold properties of foods. You do not want to put a food with too extreme a temperature in our bodies because this temperature interferes with optimal digestion. If you have a food that is cold, it can impede movement in your intestines and cause loose stools. For example, if for breakfast you are having cereal with soy milk and fruit, then I would suggest also having a cup of hot tea with it or right after your meal to help digest the cold food more efficiently. I recommend this because the soy milk is cold and the fruit (depending on which kind of fruit), which is usually not cooked and contains natural sugar, can slow digestion. You need a warm part of your meal to balance out the cold elements of your meal.

Next, TCM looks at the "flavors" of foods. These are not the actual taste that a food has when you eat it, but the characteristic properties and actions it has on your body and energy. The five flavors are sweet, bitter, sour, salty, and spicy. Each of these flavors is associated with a specific meridian. Foods play an important role in how the meridians function in the body.

The flavors of foods are also influential during the seasons of the year. The Chinese believe that the seasons have a significant effect on development and well-being. In TCM we recommend certain foods according to their flavor during certain seasons because actions of those foods can enhance health during those seasons. For one reason, we want you to eat foods when they are in season because those foods are what your body needs at the time of year those

foods are grown. It is amazing how nature grows the foods you need for nourishment according to the time of year! The nutrients and vitamins you need
are already provided in the foods. For example, if you look at root vegetables
which are grown in the fall and winter, you can see they are more warming and
nourishing during the cold times of year. It is also amazing how nature grows
certain foods for the specific environment and temperatures you live in. In
tropical or subtropical regions, for instance, citrus fruits and other foods that
are cooling for your body are grown. These cooling foods are optimal for those
living in a warmer climate.

Promoting Efficient Digestion

Along with making food choices according to TCM recommendations, it's important to pay attention to your digestion. Efficient digestion allows your body
to absorb all of the nutrients it takes in through food and supplements. You can
make digestion easier for your body by using a few guidelines. First, avoid and/
or limit raw, uncooked foods. It is okay to occasionally enjoy raw foods during
the summertime or in warmer climates where your body is already warm, but
it is best not to have uncooked foods during the wintertime or in a cold climate.

Another important part of digestion is to chew your food thoroughly and
slowly. The first step in digestion occurs when you chew your food. When you
consume a meal, your qi moves to the digestive area of your body to quickly do
its job for digestion. But if you have to eat quickly and/or stand up while eating,
this action burdens your digestive process; it is taxing on your system and can
leave you feeling sluggish. By eating slowly, you give your digestive tract the
time it needs to move everything as it should and allows you to feel your "full"
signal, which includes being mindful while you eat. Be aware of the wonderful
flavors, aromas, textures, and tastes of the foods you eat.

Eating Is About More Than Nutrition

This awareness also enhances your eating experience. Your eating ritual is not
only for your fuel and nourishment but also for you to experience time with
your family and friends. You need to always enjoy your food and the entire
experience, whether you are eating by yourself on your lunch break at work or
having dinner with your family.

At this point I want to note that losing weight is not the goal of the advice in this chapter. These nutritional recommendations benefit your entire health and well-being. Although by following a plan or regimen similar to this one, you might see a reduction in your weight simply because when you begin choosing foods that are of more nutritional value, your body craves less of the non-nutrient dense foods. The more simple carbohydrates and sugars, like chips and cookies, you consume, the more you tend to crave them. The more nutrient-dense foods like grains and vegetables you consume, the more your bodies and energies desire them. You want to make healthy choices every day.

Of course, everyone indulges from time to time, and that is okay. That is part of the enjoyment of food and experiences with others—special occasions, special meals. If you constantly deprive yourself of your favorite dessert at your favorite restaurant, you might overindulge, perhaps on food we do not love so much or on "diet" foods that might have hidden sugars, artificial sweeteners, additives, and preservatives that are not good for your health for many reasons. Again, you should enjoy your food and meals with your family and friends and appreciate the experience of sharing the delicious nourishment from our beautiful earth with them.

Other Recommendations

Along with some of the recommendations I have already mentioned about foods, a few more are significant.

Organic

Try to choose as much organic food as possible. This choice is essential for your health because you want to avoid as many pesticides, additives, and preservatives in foods as possible. Although they are researched and deemed safe, you could be allergic to certain substances. Also, your reactions to these additives could be harmful to the possibility of future pregnancies.

Local

Along with organic foods, try to buy as many local foods as possible. This choice plays a role in your relationship with our immediate environment and community. The foods grown where you live are of the most nutrient value to you. By eating the most organic and local foods possible, you are supporting your digestive system. You need to always keep your digestive system and immune system working properly and efficiently! The two systems work hand-in-hand. TCM nutrition is used by the two systems in preventing disease by both building up and preserving health.

Self Care

Food choices are an important part of your lifestyle, but so is self care. This is an area that can easily be overlooked for many of us. As is mentioned in Chapter 1, as a nurse, you tend to have a lot of stress: stress from your daily "laundry list" of things to do, job-related stress, lack of sleep, family stress, relationship stress, physical stress (headache, low back pain), general worries, and concerns. All this stress can cause multiple disorders and illnesses, ranging from minor to serious: headaches, acid reflux, insomnia, irritable bowel syndrome (IBS), irregular menstrual cycles, infertility, and so on. Stress can also exacerbate an illness that might otherwise not be so extreme.

Though you have all these things on your to-do lists, you have to make time for yourself. This time is part of self awareness and self care. Carve out time for yourself and your choices. I suggest beginning with meditation. Start with 5 minutes 1–2 times a week and see how it goes. Put it on your to-do list, such as 5 minutes at the end of a meal. Then gradually increase your meditation time to 7 minutes at a time and so on. I suggest taking it slow with meditation; go at your own pace. I believe meditation is a very personal and private action, and you grow with it and learn what is best for you. Meditation, in my estimation, is vitally important because it facilitates an inner peace that you can always tap, even during your busiest days or most stressful times. That peace is always in your mind, body, and spirit; and you can always settle into it and bring calm and stillness into your day.

The more nourishing your own personal self care is, the more you have to share with your patients to help them with their own self care. They gain knowledge and awareness of their own health from you. Through self care, you give yourself even more to teach them, more than just the basic recommendation you give them to work on at home according to their individual symptoms. The more self love you have within yourself, the more you can share with those around you.

●●●●●EMPOWERING NURSES

The Nurse Becomes the Patient

"Stephanie" is a 40-year-old female patient who has been working full-time as a nurse for 15 years. She has specialized in labor and delivery for 12 years. In the beginning of her nursing career, she began working 5 days a week, about 45–48 hours a week. She is married with two children; her son is 10 years old and her daughter is 8 years old. Her husband works 55–60 hours/week. The majority of the family duties are on Stephanie's shoulders, and she works three 12-hour shifts a week. Although on her days off she is exhausted from the long shifts, she also does a majority of the household chores along with taking care of the children, all because her husband works long hours.

Although Stephanie loves her job and loves being a nurse, the schedule is taking a toll on her. She has suffered from mild insomnia on and off for the past 8 years. She falls asleep easily but wakes up throughout the night and usually has trouble falling back asleep. She has always been a worrier, always worrying about her family and friends, worrying about other people and their well-being, and finding herself easily stressed over situations. She reports occasional dizziness after a long day at work. She always has tension in her neck and shoulders—where most people hold tension and stress. Stephanie occasionally has constipation fluctuating with diarrhea. She also sweats easily without exercising, being nervous, or being active at work. She has regular menses but also has dysmenorrhea every month, which she has had her entire life, along with emotional mood swings. Stephanie feels as if her appetite is usually low, but it can fluctuate between low and normal. Her cravings tend to be toward sweets. She has a membership at her local gym but goes only about once a month because she is usually too exhausted to go or feels guilty about taking the time for herself.

One way Western medicine might analyze and diagnose Stephanie is to treat her with a sleep aid like zolpidem. From a Western standpoint, this approach could help her sleep better and accomplish more during the day (for example, work out). But zolpidem is addictive and only masks the presenting complaints. According to TCM, I would diagnose Stephanie with liver qi stagnation (presented by dizziness, tense shoulders, and dysmenorrhea); spleen qi deficiency (spontaneous sweating, constipation, and craving sweets), blood deficiency (physical duty of job, dizziness, and insomnia).

Treatment Plan

My treatment plan for Stephanie comprises the following:

- Receive acupuncture once a week for 4 weeks then re-evaluate

- Meditate everyday for at least 5 minutes, especially on a lunch break at work
- Do guided meditation before bedtime for two reasons: as something relaxing to look forward to at the end of the day and to enhance her sleep patterns
- Choose as much organic and local foods as possible
- Avoid artificial sweeteners and processed foods
- Follow these specific food recommendations: 1–2 servings (2 ounces) of red meat per week; oysters and mussels once every 2 weeks to build the blood; snacks for work to sustain energy: walnuts, brazil nuts, and almonds with dried blueberries and cranberries; fresh fruit smoothie made with hemp milk to avoid estrogens in soymilk; a decrease in coffee and an increase in green tea, as much green tea as desired; whole grains and whole grain products; salmon, cod, halibut; two servings of fruit per day; limit/avoid dairy; specific foods to nourish liver, kidney, and spleen channels—apples, beets, black beans, raspberries, spirulina, carrots, oats, and walnuts
- Aim for three meals and two snacks per day to sustain energy
- Sleep 7–8 hours per night without TV or music
- Use lavender oil with the guided meditation at bedtime to facilitate sleep
- Perform daily journaling or use a diary
- Do 5-minutes of meditation every morning
- Take lunch outside at work or eat with family in your backyard to connect with nature while enjoying your meal
- Invite friends to take walks instead of watching TV and being tempted to overindulge on a snack
- Drink 8 8-ounce glasses of filtered water per day
- Exercise three times per week: aerobic exercise to increase heart rate for 30 minutes per day and also include yoga, Tai Chi, Qigong—anything to cultivate your qi; sign up at the gym with friends for support, and you will be more likely to go consistently; change and mix up workouts often to keep from being bored; and be sure to include strength training, which is so important for women to prevent osteoporosis because weight-bearing exercises strengthen your bones and increase bone density
- Strive to get your vitamins, minerals, and nutrients from your foods rather than in supplements because they are more easily absorbed through food and it is easier for your digestion; a strong digestive system = a strong immune system = optimal health

A treatment plan like this one is not only important for Stephanie but for those around her. Following this kind of plan sets a good example for children and patients to make time for their own self care.

Make these recommendations your own. Take from them what you want and need to create your custom lifestyle. Please remember not to be overwhelmed with this information. You want to incorporate Chinese nutrition into your lifestyle. Go at your own pace by introducing new foods and recipes slowly to your food regimen. Plan your exercise goals over the next year rather than the next 2 months. Blend these new choices into your regular routines and see how easy they fit in or how you might need to adjust them so you feel comfortable. Ease into this type of nutrition regimen and make gradual choices. By taking time for yourself and your health, you can feel better every day, can have more energy, and can embrace all that life has to offer.

Discharge Care Plan

For fun, to be formally discharged from this chapter please use your prioritizing nursing skill to reinforce some of the key messages of the chapter. Place what you think would be the correct prioritized number 1-4 in order of importance next to the corresponding letter.

A. __ Incorporate meditation and/or relaxation into your daily routine every day. This creates stillness and peace in your body and mind.

B. __ TCM looks at food's properties, characteristics, flavors, and an individual's constitution when it comes to healthy nutrition.

C. __ TCM treats your entire body system, which is comprised of your mind, body, and spirit.

D. __ TCM stands for Tasty Comfort Munchies!

Congratulations! You have earned a Golden Nightingale Wing for completing the interactive portions of the chapter.

(A = 3; B = 2; C = 1; D = 4)

13

"When I inspire myself to make positive changes, I inspire others to do the same!"

–Gary Scholar

Developing Your Own Life-Support Team

Just as it takes a great team of nurses to help patients become healthier, it takes a great personal support team for you to be successful in integrating your own healthier Lifestyle Shift.

My Critical Care Support to You

I just want to seize this moment and tell you how proud I am of you for either thinking about or making a commitment to place inspiring self care, healthier nutrition, regular activity, and weight management into your daily life. I know it's not always easy for you to change your habits and behaviors to create a healthier lifestyle, but I promise it is one of the most rewarding and fulfilling actions you can do for yourself. It takes strong commitment to and compassion for yourself to succeed. Remember every day you wake up you have the power to make healthier choices for yourself. You can make the paradigm shift to a healthier lifestyle. You know you can, so the best time to start is today!

Primary Care Giver

Creating an effective support team among friends, family, co-workers, and supervisors is the difference between being successful in your healthier lifestyle efforts or not. This group of friends, family, and colleagues serves as an integrated support team encouraging and sustaining you through your efforts.

Some years ago in my own family, everyone was still eating the SAD (Standard American Diet), and it was difficult for me to participate in family functions. Now that they have made the switch to healthy lifestyles, it makes it so much easier now to participate fully with family at my sisters' homes and not have to be tempted by junk because everyone is now on the same wellness page.

My healthy lifestyle support team consists of:

1. _____
2. _____
3. _____
4. _____

An interesting point is that it's sometimes those closest to you, those with your best interest at heart, who can sabotage and push you the farthest from your healthier lifestyle goals. You've probably seen it, experienced it personally, or done it yourself. For instance, you're at a restaurant with a friend, and you try to stop eating at just the right time—not too full—but your friend says to you, "Oh, one more bite won't hurt you!" Or, a spouse/partner says, "I'm not giving up having ice cream in the refrigerator because you're trying to eat healthier!" Or a supervisor says, "It won't be any big deal for you to miss your scheduled exercise workout because I need this report done as soon as possible."

When I first got into the health and wellness field many years ago, I created a weight management and healthy lifestyle class. I would set up a meeting at the homes of my class participants to talk to their families about supporting the students' efforts in pursuing a healthier lifestyle change. I would have students explain to their family or friends the following: I am committed to living a healthier lifestyle, and I would very much appreciate your wonderful support and encouragement to help me achieve my goals. I would like to discuss with you my specific needs that would help me succeed.

Please list those things that your support team could help you with.

I feel at my best when you:

1. _____

_____

_____

2. _____

_____

_____

3. _____

_____

_____

4. _____

_____

_____

What is great about creating a support team is that when you are striving for a healthier lifestyle, you create a positive ripple effect on those closest to you for their own healthier lifestyle. I have personally and professionally witnessed the ripple effect time and again. One of the positive ripple effects you can have is modeling healthy lifestyle choices, particularly if you have children because children see through the eyes of their parents what they need to do.

Nurse Provider Duo

If you were faced with a very challenging patient, you would not hesitate to ask for another nurse's help. So apply that thought process to your own challenge of working your Lifestyle Shift. You can make your shift easier, and more fun, if you and another nurse team up to support and encourage one another in becoming healthier. You can work out together or encourage each other to eat healthier or to lose body fat percentage.

Nurse Team Up for a Cause: Wellness Challenge

Here is an example of a structured but fun way to become healthier and tap into your wonderful, giving nature.

Duration

3–6 months

Concept

Raise money for a worthy cause and at the same time give you the gift of good health.

Overview

The object of the wellness challenge is to team up with a fellow nurse and motivate each other to place fitness and healthy nutrition into their daily lives.

Create your own pledge card with your nurse partner and collect sponsor money from family and friends to be given to a charity of your choice at the end of the challenge.

Your nurse teammate not only encourages you, but also serves as your accountability partner.

- One pound of body fat loss is worth $5 (or whatever your sponsors are willing to agree to)
- Each fitness workout is worth $1
- Each healthy eating day is worth $1

You can change this challenge up as much as you want or create your own wellness challenge. You can keep track of your achievements on the honor system, or you can have your pledge card stamped when you work out at your gym, play tennis at your club, take dance classes, and so on.

Go For Your Golden Nightingale Wings

Becoming healthier is even more motivating and fun when you create an entire workplace team effort. Consider the group wellness challenge outlined in this section.

This is a fun, friendly wellness challenge that inspires every nurse to make a positive change. Nurses choose teams. The purpose of the team structure is to give each other inspiration and support and to make "Go For Your Golden Nightingale Wings" a fun experience, but the challenge can also be implemented on an individual basis if a team approach would not work in your workplace.

First, nurses are screened on four indicators of health by a clinician. Nurses are asked to complete a HIPAA (Health Insurance Portability and Accountability Act) form when they have their biometric screenings. The fifth indicator, smoking, is not screened; it is self reported.

Of the five health indicators (body fat, cholesterol, blood sugar, blood pressure, and smoking), nurses then pick two that they want to improve on or maintain within a preferred range. The Golden Wings are awarded to the team that accrues the greatest number of Golden Wings (points) over the length of the challenge. I suggest the challenge be 6 months or more because it takes at least 6 months to see a real change in cholesterol numbers.

Golden Nightingale Wing Points

As indicated earlier, each nurse chooses two of the five health indicators to improve on or maintain as part of the challenge. Points are based upon successfully maintaining within a preferred range or improving on the two health indicators the employee has chosen.

You award 50 Golden Nightingale Wings for:

- Improving each of the two health indicators chosen as goals

- Maintaining results already in the preferred range, if the nurse made this their goal

●●●●●EMPOWERING NURSES

Health Indicators	Preferred Range:
Body fat %	Women 32% or below
	Men 25% or below
Total Cholesterol	Less than 200 mg/dl
or use	
HDL	Women greater than 50 mg/dl
	Men greater than 40 mg/dl
LDL	Less than 100 mg/dl
Blood Sugar	Less than 100 mg/dl
Blood Pressure	Less than 120/80 mm/Hg
Smoking	Quit smoking for the duration of the challenge (honor system)

Bonus Golden Nightingale Wing Points

At the end of the challenge, you award 10 bonus Golden Nightingale Wing points for maintaining results (within the preferred range) or improving the results on each of the three remaining indicators that were chosen as goals for a possible additional total of 30 bonus points awarded.

Award nurses one additional Golden Nightingale Wing point each time they participate in an eligible activity to encourage the use of fitness centers, sports facilities, or wellness programs. You can track the teams through sign-in sheets.

An alternative option is to award nurses a Golden Nightingale Wing point for reaching a specific goal in nutrition, fitness, or self care that's monitored by a wellness coach or an accountability partner.

Biometric Screening: Re-screen after 6 Months or More

- Health indicators are re-screened.
- Golden Nightingale Wing point totals are calculated.

Awards Ceremony

- Awards are presented. The importance of the award ceremony is to provide the participants with the feeling of recognition, validation, and accomplishment for all their wonderful effort to incorporate healthier lifestyles into their daily lives.

Alternative Challenge 1

If you do not want to implement the biometric screenings, you can award Golden Nightingale Wing points per day in various other ways, for example:

- Eating healthy and portion-sized meals or snacks: 1 Golden Nightingale Wing point awarded for a healthy and portion-sized meal or snack, so 3 meals plus 2 snacks = 5 Golden Nightingale Wing points per day

- Performing 30 minutes of fitness a day = 10 Golden Nightingale Wing points

- Losing 1 pound or more per week =10 bonus Golden Nightingale Wing points

- Achieving a personal self care goal for the week (getting a massage, enacting boundary setting, and so on) = 10 bonus Golden Nightingale Wing points

Alternative Challenge 2

I Bet I Can Plan is simply a fun challenge where you bet on yourself on a daily basis to eat healthier food and portion sizes and to exercise. You can implement this challenge only with yourself or with a friend or co-worker.

The currency you use is Nightingale Wellness Bucks. You bet yourself $10 Nightingale Wellness Bucks for each successful day you incorporate eating healthy or exercising. If you are successful for that day, you win $10 Nightingale Wellness Bucks. You also receive a bonus of $10 Nightingale Wellness Bucks for each pound you lose. The goal is to win $70 worth of Nightingale Wellness Bucks or more a week. Your extrinsic reward can be whatever you choose. It can be buying yourself a massage or going out for a nice healthy meal. Your intrinsic reward is the satisfaction that you're raising your quality of life and giving yourself a soft place to land—a time for a nurse to be assertive and create a healthy boundary of time that focuses on her own self care as a priority—15 minutes or more of "me" time that you can use to reflect inwardly, giving yourself positive strokes for reaching your goal.

Support Nurses Time and Energy

Talk to your administrator about providing nurses with a personal concierge service that might help ease the stress and time commitment for nurses' personal responsibilities and chores. A hospital companion program for patients and families (http://www.hospitalcompanions.com/) might also benefit nurses, freeing up time and energy spent now on support between families and patients.

Honor the Nurse Hero Within

You are the hero to so many people—hundreds, thousands, even millions, maybe—including grandparents, dads, moms, brothers, sisters, and children. Your compassionate smile, your unending support, and your professional expertise make us feel reassured and comforted when we feel hopeless and vulnerable. You care for all our needs when we need it the most. You treat your patients like one of your family. You add your sense of humor when laughter is the only thing that can help us get through the day. Not only do you deserve our undying thanks, but we ask you to take the time and energy for yourself to live well. Honor our hero by nurturing first the hero within you.

> May your Nightingale Wings not only spread in helping us, but may they help you soar to a new level of self care and living well!
>
> –Gary Scholar

Discharge Care Plan

For fun, to be formally discharged from this chapter please use your prioritizing nursing skill to reinforce some of the key messages of the chapter. Place what you think would be the correct prioritized number 1-4 in order of importance next to the corresponding letter.

A. __ Creating a support team is essential in living a healthier lifestyle.

B. __ Teaming up with a nurse partner is an effective way to get you kick-started in implementing a healthier lifestyle.

C. __ Creating an entire team of nurses to support and encourage one another is a successful plan to create a healthier lifestyle.

D. __ Great support is lying on a comfy couch with a pint of mint chocolate chip ice cream to attain a healthy amount of TV watching.

Congratulations! You have earned a Golden Nightingale Wellness Wing by completing the interactive portions of the chapter!

(A = 1; B = 3; C = 2; D = 4)

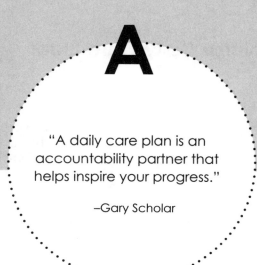

A

"A daily care plan is an accountability partner that helps inspire your progress."

–Gary Scholar

Personalizing Your Assertive Nurse Daily Care Plan

Here you will chart your fitness, nutrition, and self care functions. This is an assessment of your plans and outcomes, but also a record of how assertive you have been in acting for your own best interests and well-being. This charting process will help you with self accountability and awareness.

Assertive Nurse Daily Care Plan

Charting Nutrition

Fill in the diagram of Energy Plate Portion Size ¼ protein, ¼ whole grains, ½ veggies or fruits for breakfast, lunch, and dinner. For example; if you ate a breakfast consisting of egg whites, rye toast, and a grapefruit then write in egg whites in the protein portion section, rye toast in the whole grain portion section, and grapefruit in the fruit portion section. Or, if you ate a dinner of fish, brown rice, and green beans, write in fish in the protein portion of the plate, brown rice in the whole grain portion section, and green beans in the veggie portion section. Fill out a plate for each meal.

	Plan	**Actual Outcomes**

Day 1/Date: _____

Breakfast: _____   _____

Snack: _____   _____

Lunch: _____   _____

Snack: _____   _____

Dinner: _____   _____

	Plan	**Actual Outcomes**

Day 2/Date: _____

Breakfast: _____ _____

Snack: _____ _____

Lunch: _____ _____

Snack: _____ _____

Dinner: _____ _____

Day 3/Date: _____

Breakfast: _____ _____

Snack: _____ _____

Lunch: _____ _____

Snack: _____ _____

Dinner: _____ _____

Day 4/Date: _____

Breakfast: _____ _____

	Plan	Actual Outcomes

Snack: _____ _____

Lunch: _____ _____

Snack: _____ _____

Dinner: _____ _____

Day 5/Date: _____

Breakfast: _____ _____

Snack: _____ _____

Lunch: _____ _____

Snack: _____ _____

Dinner: _____ _____

Day 6/Date: _____

Breakfast: _____ _____

Snack: _____ _____

Lunch: _____ _____

	Plan	Actual Outcomes
Snack:	_____	_____
Dinner:	_____	_____

Day 7/Date: _____

Breakfast:	_____	_____
Snack:	_____	_____
Lunch:	_____	_____
Snack:	_____	_____
Dinner:	_____	_____

Weight Management

Body Fat Percent:	_____	_____
or		
Clothes Size:	_____	_____

Personal Self Care (massage, boundary setting, etc.):

_____   _____

_____   _____

Energy Level 1–10 (1 is low and 10 is high)

Energy Level: _____

LIVEWELL

Write to Lose

According to the *American Journal of Preventive Medicine* (2008), the most powerful predictors of weight loss are food diaries. Those who kept a food diary lost about twice as much as those who didn't keep one.

Awarded Nightingale Wings

At the end of each day check off the Nightingale Wings you have attained in nutrition, fitness, weight management, or personal self care

I am extremely proud of myself for achieving my:

_____ **GOLDEN NIGHTINGALE WINGS** - achieved my daily goal in three of the four categories

_____ **SILVER NIGHTINGALE WINGS** - achieved my daily goal in two of the four categories

_____ **BRONZE NIGHTINGALE WINGS** - achieved my daily goal in one of the four categories

Fitness Nurse Daily Care Plan
Date: _____

Strength Training

Upper Body	Exercise	Reps	Sets
1. _____	_____	_____	_____
2. _____	_____	_____	_____
3. _____	_____	_____	_____
4. _____	_____	_____	_____
5. _____	_____	_____	_____
6. _____	_____	_____	_____

Lower Body			
1. _____	_____	_____	_____
2. _____	_____	_____	_____
3. _____	_____	_____	_____
4. _____	_____	_____	_____
5. _____	_____	_____	_____
6. _____	_____	_____	_____

Aerobic (walking, jogging, swimming, biking, etc.)

Exercise	Duration	Distance
1. _____	_____	_____
2. _____	_____	_____

Fitness & Relaxation (Tai Chi, Yoga, Pilates, etc.)

1. _____
2. _____

Fun (sports, dance, ice skating, etc.)

1. _____
2. _____

Empowered Fitness (nature hike, kayaking, snorkeling, etc.)

1. _____
2 _____

Inspired Nurse Self Care Certificate

Golden Nightingale Wings

Living Well Award

Presented to

_____
(Name)

_____
(Date)

Sigma Theta Tau International
Honor Society of Nursing®

"Reading food labels is just as important as reading a patient's chart. They both are important tools to improve health!"

–Gary Scholar

Staging Your Own Food Shopping Intervention: Strategies for Navigating Those Dangerous Aisles

Food shopping is the first intervention to eating healthier. Many grocery stores contain nearly 50,000 food options. Eating healthier starts with making assertive choices that support your health, energy, and Lifestyle Shift. The shopping care plan provided here will give you the necessary knowledge to stage your own healthy food intervention.

As a nurse, you are educated in the proper procedure on how to read charts pertaining to your patients. Reading a food label is also instrumental to charting your choices in a grocery store. Because your hectic schedule creates time constraints, you can use the speed-reading guideline I've provided here to help you read a food label in only a few seconds and make assertive, healthy choices.

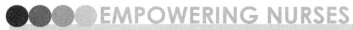 EMPOWERING NURSES

My Healthy Food Label Guidelines

For a speed read of the amount of sugar in your food or drink, you only have to focus on the sugar line and the ingredient descriptions.

Names of sugar that can fool you while reading the ingredients on a food label: Corn sweetener, corn syrup, high fructose corn syrup, dextrose, fructose, glucose, lactose, maltose, sucrose, honey, brown sugar, invert sugar, molasses, malt syrup, syrup. Definition of added sugars: during preparation or processing the sugars added to the food or drink.

Sugars that occur naturally: Found in whole fruit and vegetables are healthier then added sugar because of the added benefits of the whole foods.

Guide to Reading Food Labels:

Serving Size: Check to see if the serving size you consume is the amount considered a serving by the manufacturers. Most times what you end up eating far exceeds the one serving size on the package. Know how much you are eating so that you can use the food label to identify calorie, fat, sugar, fiber, and sodium amounts accurately.

Saturated Fat & Trans Fat: Limit foods that have saturated fat or trans fat because they raise your risk of heart disease.

Cholesterol: Try to limit your cholesterol intake to 200 mg per day or less. Cholesterol can raise your risk of heart disease.

Sodium: Try to keep your sodium intake to 1,200 mg or less per day if you have high blood pressure or a family history of high blood pressure. Remember 1 teaspoon of salt from the salt shaker has about 2,400 mg of sodium. Choose less processed foods to reduce intake.

Fiber: If meeting fiber recommendations of 20-25 grams per day is a goal. Then look for foods that have a minimum of 2-3 grams of fiber per serving. Whole fruits, vegetables, and whole grains are good sources of fiber. The higher in fiber foods tend to be lower in overall calories.

Sugars: If you are buying sweets or processed foods and beverages, then choose those that contain 4-6 grams per serving or less of added sugar. No more then 10% should come from added sugars per day.

For example, an individual eating 2,000 calories per day should not eat more than 25 grams of added sugar daily on a regular basis. Unfortunately, the average person in the U.S. will consume over 22 teaspoons of added sugar per day. Choose foods and beverages that show any added sugar as the fourth ingredient or below in the ingredient list.

Ingredient List: Will provide you with identifying what ingredients are contained in the product by weight. Choose foods or beverages that show any added sugars as the fourth ingredient or below. Also "partially hydrogenated" and "hydrogenated" are unhealthy trans fats.

Nutrition Facts

Serving Size: Serving size could be very small (4 potato chips) to make it appear that the food is low in calories, sodium, or fats.

Servings Per Container: Gives you the true picture when you eat the entire bag.

Amount Per Serving

Calories: Multiply the calories times servings per container to understand the real calorie picture.

Percent of daily value based on 2,000 calories gives you a quick picture if food has large or small amount of the nutrient.

Total Fat

Saturated Fat: 20 grams or less per day

Trans Fat: 0 per day

Cholesterol: 150 milligrams or less per day

Sodium: 1,200 milligrams or less per day

Total Carbohydrate

Dietary Fiber: 20–25 grams per day

Added Sugars: 4–6 grams or less per serving

No more than 10% of your daily diet should come from added sugar. For example, an individual eating 2,000 calories per day should not eat more then 25 grams of added sugar daily on a regular basis.

Ingredients

Choose foods that have sugar, honey, high fructose corn syrup, dextrose, and/or molasses, etc. as the fourth ingredient or lower.

Nutritional Measurements

1,000 milligrams = 1 gram

5 grams = 1 teaspoon

28 grams = 6 teaspoons = 1 ounce

Healthy Comfort-Food Shopping

Now that you can speed read a food label to identify what is healthy for you, commit to buying three or more healthy comfort foods you have never tried before. Half of them you aren't going to like and will never try again, and half of them you are going to love. Within a few months you will have new healthy comfort food options that you can enjoy!

LIVEWELL

Local Foods

Many communities have embraced the concept of fresh, local food—either directly from farmers who offer community supported agriculture (CSA) subscriptions or through farmers markets. When you buy your produce directly from a farmer, you can know more about how it was grown and harvested. Not only that, but it is typically harvested within only hours of your purchase, ensuring optimal nutrition. Find your local food options through www. localharvest.org.

Chart Your List

Before you shop, chart a list of meals and snacks for your upcoming week's schedule. Plan ahead. By doing so you invest time in the front end, so it reduces your stress on the back end. So when Thursday night rolls around, you have healthy choices in your home. Say goodbye to the need to grab fast food because you have nothing at home.

Approximately two-thirds of your grocery store purchases might be impulse buys. If you shop when you're hungry, your impulses are amplified. Everything looks delicious when you're hungry! You spend more money, and you impulse buy unhealthy comfort foods. So make sure you make healthier choices by shopping on a comfortably full stomach and make a grocery list before you leave home. If you are a bargain shopper, use your list to look for coupons (online or through your local newspaper) or sales to save you significant money.

Surgical Power Shopping

Shop around the perimeter of your grocery store in a surgical fashion by choosing "Code Emerald" foods—wonderful gems of energy-dense, high-performance foods such as veggies, fruits, whole grains, fish, lean meats, and legumes. Remember, grocery stores are designed to encourage you to spend as much money as possible. Keep that in mind, and it will be easier to resist temptations and save you calories in addition to money.

Examples of Emerald Foods: Jump Start your Health

WHOLE GRAINS:

- brown and wild rice
- whole wheat pasta
- sweet potato
- legumes, squash, yams

VEGETABLES:

- artichokes
- asparagus
- bok choy
- collard greens
- Swiss chard
- spinach
- zucchini
- beans, green and yellow

FRUITS

- apples
- blueberries
- cherries
- peaches
- pears
- prunes

NUTS & SEEDS

- almonds
- walnuts
- pumpkin, sesame, sunflower seeds

COLDWATER FISH

- wild salmon
- sardines
- wild halibut
- wild haddock
- cod
- sea bass

MEATS

- free range chicken
- free range turkey
- free range wild gamey meats
- lean beef

LIVEWELL

Paying for Calories Through Your Nose
Ever notice that fresh-baked bread (or cakes or pastries) smell when you walk into the grocery store? The bakery and deli sections are strategically placed near the entrance to most grocery stores to lure you with the scents. A full stomach will help you resist temptation.

Produce

The first Code Emerald foods you typically encounter in a grocery store are in the produce section. Fruits and vegetables are high in nutritional benefits and low in calories. Look for produce in season because it is at its richest in flavor and nutrition and is less expensive as well. Remember to try some fruits and vegetables you have never tried before!

LIVEWELL

Picking Produce
Buy produce during the week because most deliveries are Monday through Friday. Also, reach to the back or top to buy the freshest.

If you're following the healthy food portion plate, then 25% of your shopping purchases should be for proteins such as lean meats, chicken, turkey, fish, and so on; 25% should be whole grains; and 50% of weekly purchases should be vegetables and fruits.

Bakery

The next stop is the bread section. Look for breads that have a whole grain or whole grain flour listed as the first ingredient on the food label. You can buy whole grain pastas, brown rice, and bulgur for portion-controlled side dishes.

Seafood

Next you come to the fish section. Cold water fish like wild salmon, halibut, sardines, and tuna provide Omega 3 fatty acids for brain and heart health and protein to sustain energy levels and satisfy hunger.

LIVEWELL

Mercury in Fish?

A lot has been written about mercury in fish. If you're concerned, don't just avoid fish. WebMD has a good overview of this topic, including many good tips. Search for "mercury in fish" at the WebMD site or go to http://www.webmd.com/food-recipes/tc/avoiding-mercury-in-fish-topic-overview.

Meat

You next stop is the meat section. The operative word here when looking for meat is *lean*. Also remember portion control.

If you choose to consume lean meat at a meal, it should count as the 25% protein portion of your meal, which leaves 25% for whole grains and 50% for vegetables or fruit.

Red meats which include beef, pork, and lamb have high concentrations of iron but also have high concentration of unhealthy saturated fats. If you choose lean cuts coming from the loin portion of the animal the saturated fat content decreases. When consuming chicken or turkey it is recommended to use breast meat when possible and take off the skin.

- Select lean meat cuts and cut off visible fat before cooking.

- Cook skinless cuts of poultry meat.

- Try to buy organic or from your local farmers whenever possible. This way you can know or find out what the animals were fed.

- Eat less! Try making some of your meals meat-free and when you do eat meat, try smaller portions.

- Use marinades. Marinades tenderize meat and keep it moist while cooking. They also can enhance flavor that may be lost when you trim fat. Choose low-fat marinades, such as mixtures of herbs or spices with wine, low-sodium soy sauce, or lemon juice.

- Low-fat cooking methods include grilling, broiling, roasting, sautéing, and baking.

LIVEWELL

Beef: Grass- or Corn-fed?

According to WebMD, look for grass-fed beef. "Beef from grass-fed cattle is leaner, lower in fat and calories, while higher in vitamin E16 and antioxidants than beef from cattle raised on a corn diet. It is also lower in saturated fats and higher in Omega 3 fats. One study showed eating grass-fed beef helped reduce 'bad' cholesterol and increased 'good' cholesterol. Cattle raised on pasture rather than on corn-based diets also may be less susceptible to contamination with E. coli and other disease-causing bacteria" (2009, ¶ 3).

Deli

A quick trip to the deli counter helps make lunch and dinner more convenient. When possible, steer clear of bologna, salami, liverwurst, and other processed high-fat meats. They will be high in saturated fat, cholesterol, and sodium. Turkey, chicken, lean ham, and roast beef are now available in most delis in low-fat and lower sodium versions. If you want help with portion control, have the deli employee slice all your meats in 1 ounce servings so you know exactly what you are putting in your sandwich. Also look for lite tuna salad and lite chicken salad alternatives. Look for reduced fat versions of natural cheeses. Take advantage of having these sliced in 1 ounce amounts also. Look for vinai-grette salads and avoid the mayonnaise or salad dressing coated options. Many salads are now available with whole grains like brown rice and bulgur which increases your fiber intake for the day.

Inner Aisles

Now you have to leave the perimeter of the store. Here are a few tips to help you navigate the pitfalls.

Oils

A Doctor's Kitchen, a blog by Deborah Chud, MD, has a nice chart of various oils (http://www.adoctorskitchen.com/about/building-blocks). In general, look for oils high in monounsaturated fats, low in saturated fats, and avoid anything that has trans fats.

Salad Dressings

Picking a salad dressing can be tricky. Many dressings are loaded with fats or sugars. One dressing might be fat free but high in sodium, and another might be low in sodium, but high in sugar and calories. Consider retraining your taste buds and going for a sprits of fresh lemon juice or a balsamic vinegar instead of a prepared dressing. Get your other salad flavors through your choice of vegetables, fruits, and nuts and seeds.

Canned Goods

Avoid canned foods—except beans and soups—whenever possible. Vegetables are best used fresh or frozen so they maintain most of their nutritional values. Dried or canned beans can provide iron and fiber. Don't forget to check the labels! Canned goods typically contain a lot of sodium. Rinse your canned beans before using them, so they won't be as slimy. Try almond butter full of protein, fiber, and healthy monounsaturated fats. When choosing a canned soup, look for those that are broth based, contain vegetables and beans, and come in a reduced sodium version. Remember canned soups usually have 2 servings per can. So you double the amount of sodium if you consume the entire can (750 milligrams of sodium per serving suddenly become 1,500 milligrams of sodium).

Rice and Pastas

To keep your blood sugar level and fill you up so you don't overeat you should look for brown or wild rice and whole wheat pasta.

Prepackaged Foods

Avoid them like the plague. If you have to use them, do so sparingly and with a keen eye on the nutritional data. One of the unhealthiest ingredients in prepackaged foods is hydrogenated oil.

Cereals

Next, you can move up the cereal aisle. Pick low-sugar cereals that are 6 grams or lower per serving, and the fourth ingredient or lower of sugar, honey, and so on. They typically reside on the top shelf. Better yet, go for the really good breakfast grains—steel-cut oats, old fashioned oats (avoid the "instant" as they lack a lot of the nutrition and fiber, and the long cooking doesn't really take that long), cream of wheat, cream of rye, cream of buckwheat. Try an informal test with whole grains. Eat your regular cereal one morning and track how you feel, at what point you get hungry, and so on. The next day try old fashioned oatmeal to see if you don't feel fuller longer into the morning with more stable blood sugars.

Frozen Foods

I hope you're dressed warm because it's time to make a quick stop at the frozen food section. You find frozen vegetables, fruits, and whole grain waffles here. Just put on blinders as you pass by the ready made meals, frozen pizzas, ice cream, and white bagels. Stay away from anything that's breaded, and keep your eye on the nutritional data!

Dairy

Next, you head to the dairy section. I'm not a big fan of dairy products, because they can contain unhealthy amounts of saturated fats, cholesterol, antibiotics, hormones, and it creates a buildup of mucous for those that have sinus issues or it can create bloating and discomfort for those who are lactose intolerant. If you choose to use dairy, look for the 1% fat or less skim milk. Better yet, choose organic milk, which does not contain antibiotics or synthetic growth hormones. Soy milk or rice milk is another alternative. Vanilla soy milk usually has a little more added sugar than plain soy milk, so be sure to check the label. When choosing yogurt, watch out for the varieties that have 28 grams or so of added sugar per serving. The best idea is to buy a no-sugar yogurt and add your own healthy fruit to it. (If berries are not in season, you can buy frozen blueberries or mixed fruits and mix them into your no-sugar plain yogurt.) Look for reduced fat or skim versions of natural cheeses.

Bypass Surgery

Avoid the "Code Blue" foods—cookies, snack cakes, chips, sodas, and so on. You can use the Pet Supplies aisle or the Household Cleaners aisle as an alternative route to bypass many temptations. Besides, you can always use food for your beloved pet or a nice, soft, and double-ply roll of toilet paper!

LIVEWELL

Code Blue Foods

Code Blue foods are anything that's not healthy (and could well contribute to premature death)! Imagine a giant "Code Blue" sign over the chips and sodas aisles. When you start to reach for those gooey sticky buns, imagine a giant "Code Blue" stamp on the package. Tempted to grab a TV dinner? Wait, that says "Code Blue" instead of Salisbury Steak!

Saving More Than Money

"You are what you eat" is more than just a slogan. Author, editor, and food activist, Michael Pollan, points out that, "It is no coincidence that in this period when our health care costs were going from 5% of our income to 18% [1960-2009], our spending on food was plummeting from 16% to now under 9%" (Pollan, 2009). Good food doesn't have to be expensive, but it needs to be healthy. Use your critical, surgically precise shopping skills to get the best foods possible for your health and wellness and start to see the difference high quality foods make in your energy and overall health.

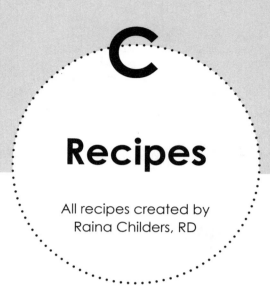

Recipes

All recipes created by
Raina Childers, RD

Appetizers and Snacks

Five-Pepper Hummus

Hummus is an easy and healthy appetizer served as a dip for vegetables, baked pita chips, or baked tortilla strips. This fresh, spicy alternative is fun when served right from a bell pepper "dish" and can be made ahead to allow the flavors to meld. The moisture from the banana peppers allows for the omission of olive oil.

1 large green bell pepper

1 can (15.5 ounces) garbanzo beans, drained

4 fresh jalapeno peppers

1 jar (16 ounces) banana peppers, drained

1 clove garlic

2 teaspoons, ground cayenne pepper

2 tablespoons ground black pepper

¼ cup tahini

Remove top ¼ of the green bell pepper, keeping bottom part intact for use for serving the hummus. Discard the stem and remove the seeds and pulp from both parts of the pepper.

Chop the top part of pepper. In a food processor or blender, combine the chopped bell pepper, garbanzo beans, jalapeno peppers, banana peppers, garlic, cayenne pepper, black pepper, and tahini. Blend into a smooth paste. Scoop the hummus into bottom part of the green bell pepper and chill.

Serves 16

Serving Size: 2 tablespoons, Calories: 63, Fat: 2.5 grams, Sodium: 107 mg, Carbohydrate: 8.9 grams, Protein: 2.3 grams

Southwest Snack Mix

This spicy, crunchy snack mix is perfect for a party or lunchbox. The almonds and dried cranberries make it satisfying and just a little sweet.

1 tablespoon canola oil

2 tablespoons lime juice

½ teaspoon chili powder

2 cups toasted high-fiber corn cereal or crispy corn and rice cereal

1 cup small pretzel knots

½ cup whole almonds

¼ cup dried cranberries

In a large skillet, heat oil over medium heat, then add lime juice and chili powder and cook for 30 seconds. Add cereal, pretzels and almonds. Cook for 4-6 minutes or until cereal and almonds are lightly browned, stirring frequently. Remove from heat and stir in dried cranberries. Spread snack mix on a baking sheet to cool.

Serves 6

Serving Size: ½ cup, Calories: 125, Fat: 7 grams, Sodium: 133 mg, Carbohydrate: 16 grams, Protein: 3 grams

Baked Tortilla Strips

When baked, flour tortillas make the perfect snack. These chips are good with hummus and also as a garnish to the Chicken Tortilla Soup.

3 whole grain flour tortillas, 8 inch

Olive oil mist or cooking spray

Preheat oven to 350 degrees. Slice tortillas into strips 3 inches long by ½ inch wide. Spray strips with cooking spray. Bake for 10 minutes until crisp.

Serves 6

Serving Size: ½ tortilla, Calories: 72, Fat: .5 grams, Sodium: 165 mg, Carbohydrate: 13 grams, Protein: 2 grams

Soups

Chicken Tortilla Soup

This flavorful and filling soup is easy to prepare and freezes well. It is best when topped with baked tortilla strips or avocado.

1 tablespoon olive oil

1 medium yellow onion, chopped

1 tablespoon garlic, minced

1 pound chicken breast, cooked

2 cans (14.5 ounces) diced tomatoes with green chilies

2 cans (6 ounce) of tomato paste

6 cups reduced sodium chicken broth

1 tablespoon cumin

Salt and pepper to taste

Heat olive oil in a large pot over medium heat, then add the onion and garlic cooking and stirring frequently until the onion becomes translucent. Add the shredded chicken breast, canned tomatoes and chilies, tomato paste, and chicken broth to the pot and stir until thoroughly mixed. Add cumin. Bring soup to a boil and then cover and reduce heat to a simmer for 15-20 minutes. Season with salt and pepper.

Serves 6

Serving Size: 2 cups, Calories: 285, Fat: 13 grams, Sodium: 600 mg, Carbohydrate: 16 grams, Protein: 22 grams

Chunky Sausage, Corn, and Habanero Chili

Habaneros are known as one of the hottest chilis around. If you're looking for something a little less spicy, try ancho or jalapeno peppers. This thick spicy stew is perfect served over rice.

1 ¼ cups prepared salsa

1 red bell pepper, diced (about 1 cup)

1 yellow bell pepper, diced (about 1 cup)

2 teaspoons chili powder

1 can (15.5 ounce) whole kernel corn, drained or 2 cups fresh or frozen corn

¼ cup habanero peppers, seeds removed

1 ½ cups smoked turkey or chicken sausage, cooked, or 1 ½ cups chicken, cooked and cut into ½ inch pieces

2 cups long grain rice, cooked

¼ cup fresh cilantro, chopped

¼ cup light or fat free sour cream

Combine salsa, bell peppers, chili powder, corn, habanero peppers, and meat in a large stock pot over medium heat. Bring to a boil, then reduce heat and simmer for 30-40 minutes. To serve, place ½ cup of rice into each bowl; top each serving with 1 cup chili. Garnish with 1 tablespoon of cilantro and 1 tablespoon of sour cream.

Serves 4

Serving Size: 1 cup chili mixture over ½ cup rice topped with 1 tablespoon sour cream and 1 tablespoon cilantro, Calories: 395, Fat: 8 grams, Sodium: 900 mg, Carbohydrate: 63 grams, Protein: 18 grams, Fiber: 9.5 grams

Squash-Quinoa Soup

Quinoa (pronounced keen-wah) is a whole grain native to South America. It is known for its mild, nutty flavor and quality protein content. It is usually found in the rice and pasta areas of the grocery store.

2 teaspoons olive oil

¾ pound of skinless, boneless chicken breasts, halved, cut into 1-inch pieces

⅓ cup onion, finely chopped

2 cans (14 ounce) reduced-sodium, low-fat chicken broth, about 3½ cups

⅓ cup apricot or mango nectar

1 pound butternut squash, peeled, halved, seeded, cut into 1-inch pieces and blanched

¾ cup dry quinoa, rinsed and drained

1 teaspoon cumin

2 small zucchini, about 5-6 ounces, halved lengthwise and cut into 1-inch pieces

Salt and pepper to taste

In large soup or stock pot, heat oil over medium heat, then add the chicken and onion. Cook and stir over medium heat for 2-3 minutes. Add chicken broth, apricot nectar, butternut squash, quinoa and cumin. Bring to boiling; reduce heat. Cover and simmer for 5 minutes. Add zucchini. Cover and cook 10 minutes more until squash and quinoa are tender. For a smoother soup, puree in a blender or food processor. Season with salt and pepper.

Serves 6

Serving Size: 1 1/3 cup: Calories: 226, Fat: 4 grams, Sodium: 454 mg, Carbohydrate: 31 grams, Protein: 19 grams, Fiber: 3 grams

Salads

Blackened Portobello Mushroom Salad

This spicy salad draws its flavor from a prepared Cajun seasoning mix. There are many over the counter varieties but generally, they include cayenne and black peppers, garlic powder, onion, basil, bay leaf, and a little salt.

¼ cup red wine vinegar

¼ cup balsamic vinegar

¼ cup tomato juice

1 tablespoon and 2 teaspoons olive oil

2 teaspoons Dijon mustard

2 teaspoons stone-ground mustard

¼ teaspoon ground black pepper

4 portobello mushroom caps (each about 5 inches wide)

1 tablespoon Cajun seasoning blend

12 cups gourmet salad greens

1 large tomato, cut into 8 wedges

½ cup thinly sliced red onion, separated into rings

1 can (15 ounces) cannelloni or other white beans, rinsed and drained

¼ cup crumbled reduced-fat feta cheese

In a 1-gallon, re-sealable plastic bag, combine both vinegars, tomato juice, 1 tablespoon of the olive oil, mustards, and ground pepper. Add mushrooms to the bag and seal. Marinate 10 minutes, turning occasionally. Remove mushrooms from bag and reserve marinade. Sprinkle mushrooms with Cajun seasoning. Heat remaining 2 teaspoons of olive oil in a large skillet over medium-high heat. Add mushrooms and cook for 2 minutes on each side or until very brown. Cut mushrooms diagonally into thin slices. Arrange 3 cups of salad greens on each of 4 plates. Top with mushrooms, tomato, onion rings, ¼ cup beans, and 1 tablespoon feta cheese. Drizzle marinade evenly over each salad.

Serves 4

Serving Size: 3 cups salad greens with ¼ cup beans, one quarter of mushroom mixture and 1 tablespoon feta cheese, Calories: 254, Fat: 10.7 grams, Sodium: 640 mg, Carbohydrate: 30 grams, Protein: 12.8 grams, Fiber: 6.5 grams

Citrus Chicken and Soba Noodle Salad

This tangy salad with a Japanese flair is even better with freshly-squeezed orange and lime juice. Soba noodles are made from buckwheat and are cooked like conventional pasta, but be careful not to overcook them.

1 package (8 ounces) of dried soba noodles, cooked

¾ cup carrots, cut into matchsticks

1/3 cup green onion, sliced

1 cup grape tomatoes, halved

2 tablespoons fresh cilantro

¾ pounds chicken breast, cooked, cut into 1 inch pieces

¼ teaspoon salt

¼ teaspoon black pepper

2 tablespoons orange juice

2 tablespoons lime juice

1 tablespoon low-sodium soy sauce

1 tablespoon sesame oil

After cooking, drain and place noodles in a large bowl. Add carrots, onion, tomatoes, cilantro, chicken, salt and pepper. In a separate bowl, whisk together orange juice, lime juice, soy sauce, and sesame oil. Add dressing to noodle mixture and toss well.

Serves 4

Serving Size: 2 cups, Calories: 380, Fat: 8 grams, Sodium: 850mg, Carbohydrate: 50 grams, Protein: 32 grams

Mediterranean Chicken Salad

This delicious salad is a wonderful combination of many traditional Mediterranean flavors. Orzo is a barley-shaped pasta and gives this salad texture. Capers are the cured buds off of the caper plant and are found near olives and vinegars in most grocery stores.

½ cup orzo, cooked

2 tablespoons olive oil

1 tablespoon tomato paste

2 tablespoons reduced sodium, low-fat chicken broth

3 tablespoons balsamic vinegar

1 tablespoon fresh tarragon, chopped

2 teaspoons lemon juice

2 teaspoons Dijon mustard

Black pepper to taste

3 cups chicken breast, cooked and diced

1 ½ cups cherry tomatoes, halved

1 jar (6 ounces) artichoke hearts, drained and chopped, canned would also work

½ cup kalamata or black olives, pitted and chopped

¼ cup raisins

1 ½ tablespoons capers, drained

5 cups fresh spinach leaves

4 tablespoons pine nuts, toasted

In a small bowl, whisk together olive oil, tomato paste, chicken broth, vinegar, tarragon, lemon juice, mustard, and pepper. In a large bowl, combine chicken, orzo tomatoes, artichoke hearts, olives, and capers and mix well. Drizzle dressing over top and toss. Serve each scoop of chicken salad on a bed of spinach leaves and sprinkle with pine nuts.

Serves 4

Serving Size: 1 ½ cups spinach topped with 1 cup of the chicken mixture and 1 tablespoon pine nuts, Calories: 365, Fat: 13 grams, Sodium: 700mg, Carbohydrate: 23 grams, Protein: 38 grams

Shrimp Salad with Pineapple and Pecans

This tangy twist on shrimp is delicious during warm months. The shrimp can be fresh or frozen and thawed. It is a mixture that is also yummy wrapped in a whole grain tortilla or stuffed in a whole grain pita for a complete meal.

6 ounces shrimp, shelled, deveined, cooked and cut lengthwise into halves

1 cup pineapple chunks

1 cup snow peas with stem ends removed, blanched

¾ cup pecan halves, toasted

2 tablespoons green onion, sliced

4 teaspoons low-fat mayonnaise

4 teaspoons white wine vinegar

8 cups romaine lettuce

In medium bowl, combine shrimp, pineapple, snow peas, pecans, and green onion. In a separate small bowl, whisk together mayonnaise and vinegar. Pour dressing mixture over shrimp mixture, toss and coat and let sit for about 10 minutes before serving. Place 2 cups of romaine lettuce on each plate and place shrimp mixture on top.

Serves 4

Serving Size: 2 cups romaine topped with 1 cup shrimp mixture, Calories: 250, Fat: 17 grams, Sodium: 147 mg, Carbohydrate: 15 grams, Protein: 13 grams

Jicama and Fruit Salad

The nutty, slightly sweet crunch of the jicama root gives this salad a fresh appeal especially with the kiwi fruit. If you've never worked with oddly-shaped jicama or furry kiwi fruit before, they're simple to peel with a vegetable peeler or paring knife.

1 teaspoon grated orange rind

¼ cup orange juice

2 tablespoons brown sugar

¾ teaspoon ground cinnamon

1/8 teaspoon ground nutmeg

3 cups jicama, peeled and cut into matchsticks

1 medium red grapefruit, peeled and sectioned

2 medium oranges, peeled and sliced 2 kiwi fruit, peeled and sliced

In a medium bowl, whisk together orange rind, orange juice, brown sugar, cinnamon, and nutmeg. Add jicama, grapefruit, orange slices, and kiwi fruit. Toss gently to coat.

Yield: 4 servings

Serving Size: 1 cup, Calories: 134, Fat: .5 grams, Sodium: 6 mg, Protein: 2.3 grams, Fiber: 4 grams

Spicy Asian Slaw

This cabbage slaw draws on Asian flavors instead of the mayonnaise heavy dressings found in most coleslaws. It makes a great side dish.

- ¼ cup rice wine vinegar
- 2 tablespoons low-sodium soy sauce
- 2 teaspoons sesame oil
- ¼ teaspoon crushed red pepper flakes
- ¼ cup green onions, sliced
- 1 package (16 ounce) coleslaw-cut cabbage mix
- 1 tablespoon fresh parsley, chopped
- 2 teaspoons sesame seeds, toasted

In a large bowl, whisk together vinegar, soy sauce, sesame oil, and red pepper flakes. Add green onions and the cabbage mix tossing gently to coat. Sprinkle parsley and sesame seeds on top.

Serves 4

Serving Size: 1 cup, Calories: 74, Fat: 3 grams, Sodium: 235 mg, Carbohydrate: 10.5 grams, Protein: 1.5 grams, Fiber: 2.5 grams

Springtime Fruit Salad with Citrus-Mint Dressing

Use fresh orange and lime juice along with freshly chopped mint to give this fruit salad a taste of springtime any time of year.

6 kiwi fruit, peeled and cut into wedges

2 cups honeydew melon, cubed

2 cups cantaloupe, cubed

1 medium papaya, peeled and cut into 1-inch chunks

1 tablespoon sugar or sugar-substitute

1 ½ tablespoon fresh mint, finely chopped

½ teaspoon finely grated orange peel

2 tablespoon orange juice

1 teaspoon lime juice

Combine kiwi fruit, melon, and papaya in medium bowl. In a small bowl, whisk together sugar, mint, orange peel, and juices and pour over fruit. Stir to coat and serve.

Serves 6

Serving Size: 1 ½ cups, Calories: 120, Fat: 0 grams, Carbohydrate: 29 grams, Protein: 2.5 grams

Summertime Black-Eyed Pea Salad

This bean salad has a Latin twist. It is great paired with BBQ or chicken quesa-dillas. Of course, it would also work on New Year's as well.

2 tablespoons olive oil

4 small yellow summer squash, quartered lengthwise and thinly sliced (about 4 cups)

2 jalapeno peppers, seeded and chopped

4 cloves garlic, minced

1 teaspoon cumin

2 cans (15 ounce) black-eyed peas, rinsed and drained

¼ cup green onions, sliced

2 tablespoons cilantro, chopped

¼ teaspoon salt

2 cups tomatoes, seeded, cored and chopped

In a large skillet, heat oil over medium heat. Add squash, peppers, garlic, and cumin; cook for 5-6 minutes or until squash is crisp-tender, stirring occasionally. Remove from heat; let cool. In a large bowl, combine black-eyed peas, green onions, cilantro, and salt. Add squash mixture and salt. Cover and chill. To serve, toss with fresh tomato.

Serves 8

Serving Size: ¾ cup, Calories: 160, Fat: 5 grams, Sodium: 283 mg, Carbohydrate: 24 grams, Protein: 8 grams

Vegetarian Tuscan Salad

The creamy texture and mild flavor of fresh mozzarella cheese help make this recipe a favorite anytime. Fresh mozzarella is usually sold in a liquid to keep the cheese moist. Always keep the cheese in its liquid until ready to use and then discard leftover cheese after 3 days.

5 cups spinach leaves

1 cup fresh mozzarella cheese, cubed

½ cup black olives, sliced

½ cup red onion, minced

½ cup sliced almonds, toasted

2 tomatoes, cored, seeded and chopped

1 can (15 ounces) cannellini beans, rinsed and drained

¾ cup balsamic vinegar

½ cup reduced fat feta cheese

¼ cup fresh basil, chopped

In a large bowl, combine spinach, cheese, olives, onions, almonds, tomatoes, beans, and vinegar, tossing gently to coat. Top with feta and basil; serve immediately.

Serves 6

Serving Size: 2 cups, Calories: 270, Fat: 12 grams, Sodium: 560 mg, Carbohydrate: 20 grams, Protein: 20 grams

Roasted Pepper, Wax Bean, and Tomato Salad

Roasted red bell peppers provide the centerpieces to this hearty salad perfect for late summer with fresh tomatoes and wax beans are plentiful. Don't forget, when you cook your beans, they should still have some snap!

1 medium red bell pepper, stem and seeds removed and cut in half, lengthwise	½ teaspoon salt
	2 tablespoons cider vinegar
1 pound wax beans, trimmed and cut in half	2 tablespoons lemon juice
	1 tablespoon Dijon mustard
2 cups cherry tomatoes, halved	1 ½ teaspoons sugar
½ cup green onions, sliced	1 teaspoon olive oil
¼ cup parsley, chopped	½ cup low-fat feta cheese or goat cheese

Preheat broiler. Line a baking sheet with aluminum foil. Lay bell pepper halves, skin side up on baking sheet and broil for 10 minutes or until skin begins to blacken. Remove from the oven and immediately seal peppers in a re-sealable plastic bag. Let sit 15 minutes. Remove from bag and peel skin from the pepper halves. Slice roasted peppers into strips. Bring 2 quarts water to boil. Add wax beans and boil 4 minutes until beans are crisp-tender; drain. In a large bowl, combine roasted pepper, tomatoes, onion, and parsley. In a small bowl, whisk salt, vinegar, lemon juice, mustard, sugar, and olive oil until combined. Place 1 cup of bean salad on 8 plates and drizzle with dressing. Top with feta cheese.

Serves 8

Serving Size: 1 cup, Calories: 63; Fat: 2.5 grams, Sodium: 289 mg, Carbohydrate: 8.5 grams, Protein: 3 grams; Fiber: 3 grams

Vegetables and Side Dishes

Cajun-Style Collard Greens

This spicy old school southern dish is perfect with blackened seafood or chicken. Of course paired with some red beans, rice, and smoked turkey sausage would be great too! The crushed red pepper and hot sauce can be decreased depending on what level of heat is desired.

2 tablespoons olive oil

1 yellow onion, diced

2 cloves garlic, minced

4 medium sized tomatoes, cored, seeded, and diced

¾ cup vegetable broth

1 pound collard greens, rinsed and chopped

½ teaspoon crushed red pepper flakes

½ teaspoon garlic powder

¼ teaspoon salt

¼ teaspoon black pepper

dash cayenne (optional)

½ teaspoon hot sauce (optional)

Heat oil in skillet over medium heat. Add onions and garlic. Stir and cook until onions are soft, about 5 minutes. Add vegetable broth and collard greens and cover. Cook for about 6-8 minutes, until greens are slightly soft. Add red pepper flakes, garlic powder, salt, pepper, and cayenne and hot sauce, if using. Cover and cook another 6-8 minutes, until greens are done, stirring occasionally.

Serves 8

Serving Size: 1 cup, Calories: 66, Fat: 3.5 grams, Sodium: 100 mg, Carbohydrate: 6 grams, Protein: 2.5 grams

Pine Nut Topped Green Beans

Fresh green beans are a treat, even if you're not trying to be a healthy eater. These green beans are highlighted with cured Italian ham, pine nuts, and the zing of fresh lemon.

2 teaspoons olive oil, divided

2 ounces thinly-sliced prosciutto, cut into ribbons

2 pounds green beans, ends trimmed and blanched

4 cloves garlic, minced

2 teaspoons sage, minced

¼ teaspoon salt, divided

black pepper to taste

¼ cup pine nuts, toasted

1 ½ teaspoons freshly grated lemon zest

1 teaspoon lemon juice

Heat ½ teaspoon oil in large skillet over medium heat. Add prosciutto and cook, stirring, until crispy, 4 to 5 minutes. Drain on a paper towel and set aside. Wipe out pan and heat the remaining olive oil. Add green beans, garlic, sage, 1/8 teaspoon salt, and pepper. Cook, stirring occasionally, 3-4 minutes. Stir in pine nuts, lemon zest, and the prosciutto. Season with lemon juice and the remaining salt and pepper.

Serves 8

Serving Size: 1 cup, Calories: 99, Fat: 5 grams, Sodium: 264 mg, Carbohydrate: 10 grams, Protein, 5 grams

Asparagus with Lemon and Mustard

Anything with Asparagus feels like Spring. This easy side dish has a surprising kick that many enjoy. It works well as the green vegetable for any meal but is a nice addition to a brunch menu.

24 fresh asparagus spears, trimmed

3 tablespoons fat-free mayonnaise

2 tablespoons sweet brown mustard

2 tablespoons lemon juice

2 teaspoons grated lemon peel, divided

Bring a pot of water fitted with a vegetable steamer to boil. Add asparagus, cover and steam until bright green and crisp tender–about 2-3 minutes depending on the size. In a small bowl, combine mayonnaise, mustard, and lemon juice. Stir in 1 teaspoon lemon peel. Divide asparagus between 4 servings and spoon 2 tablespoons dressing over each serving. Top with remaining lemon peel.

Serves 4

Serving Size: 6 asparagus spears and 2 tablespoons dressing, Calories: 40, Fat: 1 grams, Sodium: 294 mg, Carbohydrate: 7 grams, Protein: 3 grams, Fiber: 2gm

Basil Roasted Vegetables with Couscous

Couscous is a simple pasta alternative widely available in whole wheat and other whole grain versions. It quickly steams when you cook it and makes a great base for these roasted fall vegetables.

2 tablespoons minced fresh basil

2 tablespoons balsamic vinegar

1 tablespoon olive oil

¼ teaspoon salt

2 cloves of garlic, crushed

2 medium zucchini, cut into 1 inch pieces

1 medium red bell pepper, cut into 1 inch pieces

1 medium yellow bell pepper, cut into 1 inch pieces

1 package (8 ounce) mushrooms

3 cups hot cooked couscous

½ cup reduced fat feta or goat cheese

1/8 teaspoon pepper

Preheat oven to 425 degrees. In a large bowl, combine basil, vinegar, olive oil, salt, and garlic. Stir well, then add zucchini, bell peppers, and mushrooms. Toss well to coat the vegetables, then arrange in a single layer in a shallow roasting pan. Bake at 425 degrees for 35 minutes or until browned. Serve vegetables over couscous and top with cheese.

Serves 4

Serving Size: 1 ½ cups roasted vegetables over ¾ cup couscous and topped with 2 tablespoons feta cheese, Calories: 275, Fat: 6.4 grams, Sodium: 398 mg, Carbohydrate: 41 grams, Protein: 11 grams, Fiber: 4 grams

Vegetarian Main Dishes

Asparagus Tomato Stir Fry

This easy and low-calorie meal can be put together incredibly fast. The Asian flavors can make asparagus lovers out of even the toughest vegetable critic.

2 teaspoons cornstarch

¼ cup reduced fat low-sodium chicken broth

4 teaspoons low-sodium soy sauce

2 teaspoons minced ginger or 1 teaspoon ground ginger

1 teaspoon olive oil

¾ pound asparagus, cut into 1 inch pieces

4 green onions, cut into 1 inch pieces

1 ½ cup mushrooms, sliced

2 small plum tomatoes, cored, seeded, and cut into thin wedges

1 teaspoon sesame oil

4 cups cooked brown rice

In a small bowl, combine cornstarch, chicken broth, soy sauce, and ½ teaspoon of the ginger until blended, then set aside. Heat oil in a skillet or wok over medium-high heat. When hot, stir fry the remaining ginger for 30 seconds then add the asparagus and onions. Stir fry for 3 minutes, then add mushrooms and stir fry for 1 minute more. Stir cornstarch mixture and add to the skillet. Bring to a boil, then cook and stir for 1 minute or until thickened. Reduce heat. Add tomatoes and sesame oil, stir fry for 1 minute longer. Serve over warm brown rice.

Serves 4

Serving Size: ¾ cup of stir fry vegetables and 1 cup brown rice, Calories: 280, Fat: 5 grams, Sodium: 278 mg, Carbohydrate: 54 grams, Protein: 8 grams

Black Bean and Spinach Pizza

If pizza is a favorite, then here is a tasty recipe with a delicious Mexican vibe. The taste is so good it is hard to remember that this pizza is also good for you!

1 prepared thin pizza crust 16" or dough to prepare equivalent

1 can (15-ounce) black beans, rinsed and drained

2/3 cup onion, chopped

1 teaspoon ground cumin

1 teaspoon chili powder

1 garlic clove, minced

½ cup prepared salsa

4 cups spinach leaves

2 tablespoons cilantro, chopped

½ teaspoon hot sauce (optional)

½ cup shredded reduced fat cheddar cheese

½ cup shredded Monterey Jack cheese

Pre-bake or heat pizza crust according to package instructions. Once finished, remove and keep oven on at 375 degrees. In a medium bowl, mash beans with a fork, then add the onion, cumin, chili powder, and garlic. Combine until well mixed. Spread the bean mixture over the baked pizza crust, leaving a 1-inch border. Spoon salsa evenly over bean mixture; top with spinach and cilantro. Drizzle with hot sauce; sprinkle with cheeses. Bake at 375 degrees for 15 minutes or until crust is lightly browned. Cut pizza into 8 slices.

Serves 4

Serving Size: 2 slices, Calories: 400, Fat: 12 grams, Sodium: 900 mg, Carbohydrate: 51 grams, Protein: 22 grams, Fiber: 8 grams

Egg Fried Rice

Eggs are a wonderful base to many delicious and healthy meals. They provide excellent nutrition and are incredibly economical as well. This well-known Chinese dish can work on any day of the week and brings "take-out" home.

2 teaspoons sesame oil	1 cup frozen peas, thawed
2 whole eggs	¾ teaspoon salt
3 egg whites	½ teaspoon black pepper
1 tablespoon canola oil	1 cup bean sprouts
4 cups cold, cooked brown rice	1/3 cup chopped green onions

In a small bowl, combine sesame oil, eggs, and egg whites. Stir well and set aside. Heat oil in a large skillet or wok over medium-high heat. When the oil is hot, add egg mixture and stir fry for 2 minutes. Add rice and stir fry for 3 minutes. Add peas, salt, and pepper and stir fry for another 5 minutes. Add bean sprouts and green onions then stir fry 2 minutes and serve.

Serves 5

Serving Size: 1 cup, Calories: 240, Fat: 5.4 grams, Sodium: 348 mg, Carbohydrate: 36.4 grams, Protein: 9 grams

Artichoke Omelet

This flavor rich dish is wonderful for a weekend morning breakfast. It requires no special culinary skills, but loved ones will think hours of preparation were involved. Combine this egg delight with whole grain bread and fruit preserves.

3 cloves garlic, minced

1 cup artichoke hearts, drained, patted dry

½ cup red bell pepper, chopped

¼ cup green onions (white portion only), sliced, green portion reserved

8 kalamata or black olives, pitted and sliced

½ teaspoon dried oregano

¾ teaspoon dried basil

¼ teaspoon ground black pepper

1 carton (16 ounces) cholesterol-free real egg product

3 tablespoons grated Parmesan cheese, divided

Spray medium skillet with cooking spray; heat over medium heat. Add garlic and cook 1 minute, stirring occasionally. Add artichokes, bell pepper, onion, olives, oregano, basil, and black pepper. Cook 8 minutes, or until vegetables are crisp-tender, stirring occasionally. Remove vegetables from skillet; cover to keep warm. Keep skillet hot and add egg substitute. Once eggs are set in center, about 4-5 minutes, spoon vegetable mixture over half of omelet; sprinkle with 2 tablespoons of cheese. Slide onto serving plate and fold omelet in half. Top omelet with remaining tablespoon of cheese and green onion tops. Cut into 4 wedges to serve.

Serves 4

Serving size: 1 wedge, Calories: 121, Fat: 3 grams, Sodium 414 mg, Carbohydrate: 10 grams, Protein: 13 grams

Greek Stuffed Eggplant

Many have heard that eggplant is a healthy vegetable but are unsure of how to prepare it. This recipe's ingredients enhance the mild flavor of eggplant. It also cleverly uses as much of the mysterious purple vegetable as possible.

2 eggplants (about 3 pounds), cut in half lengthwise

¼ cup water

1 cup onion, chopped

1 cup plum tomato, cored, seeded, and chopped

¼ cup dry white wine

3 cloves garlic, minced

4 ounces reduced-fat feta cheese, crumbled

½ cup fresh parsley, chopped, divided

¾ teaspoon salt, divided

¼ teaspoon black pepper

2 slices, 1 ounce each, of French bread

2 tablespoons grated fresh Parmesan cheese

Scoop and save pulpy interior from each eggplant, reserving shells. Coarsely chop pulp to measure 6 cups and set aside. Use cooking spray to coat the inside of a 10-inch square baking dish. Place eggplant shells, cut sides down in the dish and add the water. Cover and microwave at high for 5 minutes. Remove and keep warm. In the meantime, preheat the broiler. Heat a large skillet over medium-high heat. Coat the skillet with cooking spray, and add eggplant pulp. Cook and stir 7 minutes. Add onion, cooking and stirring another 2 minutes. Stir in tomato, wine, and garlic; cook 3 minutes or until liquid is almost evaporated. Remove vegetable mixture from the heat, and add feta cheese, ¼ cup parsley, ½ teaspoon salt and pepper stirring to combine.

Coat a baking sheet with cooking spray and arrange eggplant shells face up. Spoon ¾ cup eggplant mixture into each eggplant shell. To make topping, place bread slices in the bowl of a food processor and pulse until coarse crumbs measure 1 cup. In a medium bowl, combine bread crumbs, ¼ cup parsley, ¼ teaspoon salt and Parmesan stirring well. Sprinkle ¼ cup of bread crumb mixture over each stuffed shell. Broil shells 2 minutes until browned.

Serves 4

Serving Size: 1 stuffed eggplant shell, Calories: 250, Fat: 8.4 grams, Sodium: 900 mg, Carbohydrate: 35 grams, Protein: 11.3 grams

Tofu, Asparagus, and Red Pepper Stir-Fry with Quinoa

Tofu, once considered part of the ethnic fringe, has made its way into many mainstream kitchens. Firm and extra-firm versions lend themselves to sautéing, baking, and grilling. Their dryer texture allows them to absorb the flavors of the dish and hold together through the cooking process. This heart healthy meat alternative may even make a die-hard meat eater sit up and take notice.

Dressing

2 tablespoons rice vinegar

2 tablespoons low-sodium soy sauce

2 teaspoons dark sesame oil

dash of crushed red pepper flakes

Stir-Fry

1 ½ cups water

1 ½ cups uncooked quinoa

1 tablespoon sesame oil

1 cup onion, chopped

2 cloves garlic, minced

2 cups red bell pepper, cut into strips

2 cups mushrooms, sliced

1 pound asparagus (about 2 cups) cut into 1-inch pieces

½ teaspoon salt

1 package (12.3 ounce) reduced fat firm tofu, drained and cubed

2 tablespoons sesame seeds

To make the dressing, in a small bowl, whisk together rice vinegar, soy sauce, sesame oil, and crushed red pepper flakes. Set aside. Prepare quinoa according to package instructions. Set aside. For main dish, heat sesame oil in large skillet or wok over medium-high heat. Add onion and garlic and stir-fry for 5 minutes. Add bell pepper, mushrooms, asparagus, salt, and tofu. Stir-fry for 3 minutes. Remove from heat, stir in dressing. Place ½ cup of quinoa on each plate, add vegetables and top with sesame seeds.

Serves 6

Serving Size: 1 cup stir-fry and ½ cup quinoa, Calories: 273, Fat: 8 grams, Sodium 435mg, Carbohydrate: 39 grams, Protein: 12 grams

Vegetable Pie Mexicana

A Mexican delight! Don't let the long ingredient list fool you. Assembling is easy and the results are unique and mouthwatering!

1 ½ cups green onions, sliced

½ cup green bell pepper, chopped

2 garlic cloves, minced

1 ½ cups corn, fresh or frozen

½ cup prepared salsa

2 tablespoons cilantro, minced

2 tablespoons lime juice

2 cans (15.5 ounce) pinto beans, drained

2 medium tomatoes, chopped

½ cup all-purpose flour

½ cup yellow cornmeal

½ teaspoon chili powder

1 cup skim milk

2 whole eggs, beaten

4 egg whites, beaten

1 cup shredded reduced-fat cheddar cheese

¼ cup low-fat sour cream

Preheat oven to 475 degrees. Coat a skillet with cooking spray and place over medium-high heat. Add green onions, bell pepper, and garlic. Cook and stir 3 minutes. Add corn, salsa, cilantro, lime juice, and pinto beans. Cook until heated. Remove from heat and set aside. In a medium bowl, combine flour, cornmeal, and chili powder. Gradually whisk in milk and eggs until well blended. Coat 2 pie plates (9 inch) with cooking spray. Pour half of egg mixture into one and the other half into the second pie plate. Bake both at 475 for 10 minutes or until egg base is puffed or browned. Remove from oven, and spoon half of pinto bean mixture into each pie shell over the egg base. Top with cheese. Continue baking at 475 degrees for 1-2 minutes or until cheese melts. Cut each pie into 6 pieces. Top each slice with a teaspoon of sour cream.

Serves 6

Serving Size: 2 pie wedges and 2 teaspoons sour cream, Calories: 380, Fat: 7 grams, Sodium: 520 mg, Carbohydrate: 57 grams, Protein: 25 grams

Entrees for the Meat Eaters

Asian Beef Steaks and Noodles

The garlicky, sweet taste of hoisin sauce in this recipe really makes this dish jump. Hoisin sauce is a mixture made from fermented soy and wheat and is perfect for stir-fry and marinades and you'll find it in the Asian section of your market.

1 pound beef shoulder, with fat trimmed

¼ cup hoisin sauce

1 tablespoon water

1 tablespoon red wine vinegar

¼ teaspoon crushed red pepper flakes

2 teaspoons canola oil, divided

1 ½ cups cucumbers, seeded, peeled, and sliced

1 small red bell pepper, cut into thin strips

¼ cup green onions, sliced

2 cups Chinese egg noodles, cooked and warm

1 tablespoon cilantro, chopped and divided

Cut beef shoulder into ½-1/4 inch strips. Set aside. In a small bowl, whisk together hoisin sauce, water, vinegar, and crushed red pepper flakes. Set aside. In a large skillet or wok, heat 1 teaspoon of the oil over medium-high heat until hot. Add cucumbers, bell pepper, and green onions and stir-fry 1-2 minutes until vegetables are crisp-tender. (Do not overcook.) Add cooked noodles, 1 ½ teaspoons cilantro, and half of hoisin sauce mixture; toss. Remove from skillet; keep warm. Heat remaining teaspoon of oil in same skillet. Add ½ of the beef and stir fry 2 minutes. Set cooked beef aside and repeat with second batch. Return all beef to skillet and add remaining hoisin sauce mixture; cook and stir until heated through. Place 1 cup of noodle mixture on each of four plates. Serve beef over noodles and top with remaining cilantro.

Serves 4

Serving Size: ½ cup of beef over 1 cup noodle mixture, Calories: 322, Fat: 10 grams, Sodium: 330 mg, Carbohydrate: 30 grams, Protein: 28 grams, Fiber: 2 grams

Baked Chicken Tortillas

Recreating a dish to resemble chicken enchiladas was a breeze. Not only is it yummy but it contains very little calorie consequence. Serve with a green salad and fresh melon.

1 cup prepared salsa, divided

1 container (8 ounce) fat free sour cream

6 whole wheat tortillas, 10 inch

¾ cup boneless, skinless chicken breast, cooked and chopped into ½ inch pieces

1/3 cup tomato, cored, seeded and chopped

1/3 cup green bell pepper chopped

¾ cup shredded low-fat cheddar cheese

Preheat oven to 350 degrees. In a small bowl, combine ½ cup of the salsa and the sour cream. Spread this mixture evenly over each tortilla. Place chicken, tomatoes, and green pepper down the center of each tortilla. Coat an 11x17 baking dish with cooking spray. Roll up each tortilla and place in the dish tightly, seam down. Top with ½ cup salsa. Bake at 350 degrees for 15 minutes. Sprinkle with cheese and return to oven for an additional 5 minutes or until cheese melts.

Serves 6

Serving Size: 1 filled tortilla topped with ½ cup salsa and 2 tablespoons cheese, Calories: 220, Fat: 3 grams, Sodium: 500 mg, Carbohydrate: 31 grams, Protein: 21 grams, Fiber: 3 grams

Homestyle Meatloaf

Ah, meatloaf. A true comfort food! Using lean ground beef, egg whites, and oats really bumps up this timeless favorite's nutritional value.

2 pounds beef round, ground

½ cup quick cooking oats

¼ cup onion, minced

1/8 cup green bell pepper, minced

2 large egg whites

2 tablespoons brown sugar

¼ teaspoon salt

¼ teaspoon black pepper

¾ cup ketchup, divided

Preheat oven to 350 degrees. In a large bowl, combine beef, oats, onion, bell pepper, egg whites, brown sugar, salt, pepper, and half of the ketchup. Mix well. Spray a 9-inch square baking dish with cooking spray. Shape meat into an 8-inch long loaf and place in the baking dish. Brush with the remaining ketchup. Bake at 350 degrees for 1 hour 10 minutes. Cool 10 minutes before slicing into 8 equal slices.

Serves 8

Serving Size 1 slice, Calories: 200, Fat: 8 grams, Sodium: 420 mg, Carbohydrate: 13 grams, Protein: 20 grams

Italian Chicken with Garlic and Chickpeas

A dish similar to this could be found on the table of a family in Southern Italy. It is a stove-top, one pot wonder. Dinner on a busy week-night is easy with this recipe. Serve with some crusty whole grain bread.

1 pound skinned, boned chicken thighs

¼ teaspoon salt

½ teaspoon black pepper

1 tablespoon olive oil

1 1/3 cups onion, sliced

1 cup green bell pepper, cut into strips

1 teaspoon garlic, minced

1 can (15 ounce) chickpeas, drained

1 can (14.5 ounce) diced tomatoes with basil, garlic, and oregano, undrained

¼ cup fresh, flat-leaf parsley leaves, chopped

Rinse and drain chicken, then rub meat with salt and pepper. In a large skillet, heat oil over medium-high heat. Add chicken to pan and brown, about 2 minutes on each side. Add onions and peppers. Stir and cook 4 minutes. Reduce heat to medium. Add garlic, chickpeas, and tomatoes. Cover and cook 8 minutes or until thoroughly heated and chicken is done. Top with fresh parsley.

Serves 4

Serving Size: 1 ½ cups, Calories: 370, Fat: 12 grams, Sodium: 630 mg, Carbohydrate: 28 grams, Protein: 32 grams

Pork Chops with Apple-Pear Chutney

This European style chutney combines fruit and spices creating a final product that is incredibly sweet and savory. Not only is it delicious on pork but also compliments poultry well, too. Looking for a new dessert? Don't hesitate to use the fruit part of this recipe as a topping for a low-calorie vanilla frozen yogurt or ice cream.

6 center cut pork chops, about 1-inch thick

1 tablespoon olive oil

1 teaspoon black pepper

1 cup sugar

½ cup sucralose low-calorie sweetener

1 teaspoon salt

1/8 teaspoon ground cloves

½ teaspoon ground cinnamon

1 package (12-ounce) fresh cranberries

3 pears, cored, peeled and chopped (about 2 cups)

1 Granny Smith apple, cored, peeled, and chopped (about 1 cup)

¾ cup golden raisins

1/3 cup onion, chopped

1 teaspoon ground ginger

2 tablespoons lemon juice

Preheat broiler. Lightly brush pork chops with olive oil and rub with black pepper. Set aside on a broiling pan coated with cooking spray. In a large saucepan, combine sugar, sucralose low-calorie sweetener, salt, cloves, cinnamon, and cranberries over medium heat, stirring until sugar dissolves. Reduce heat, and simmer 10 minutes or until cranberries begin to pop. Stir in pear, apple, raisins, onion, and ginger. Cook 20 minutes. Remove from heat and stir in lemon juice. Broil pork chops for 5-8 minutes each side. Top each pork chop with 2 tablespoons of the chutney and serve.

Serves 6

Serving Size: 1 pork chop with 2 tablespoons chutney, Calories: 262, Fat: 5 grams, Sodium: 125 mg, Carbohydrate: 27 grams, Protein: 21 grams

Baked Salmon with Lemon-Dill Mustard Sauce

Salmon is a wonderful source of Omega-3 fatty acids. The fresh dill and fla-vored mustard distract the palate from the stronger flavors of this healthy fish. Fish cooks quickly so keep watch to avoid a dry product.

¾ cup Dijon mustard

1 tablespoon lemon juice

1 ½ teaspoons water

4 salmon fillets, about 6 ounces each

1 ½ tablespoons fresh dill, finely chopped

½ teaspoon salt

1/8 teaspoon black pepper

Preheat oven to 350 degrees. In a small bowl, whisk together mustard, lemon juice, and water. Rinse and drain salmon filets. Brush both sides of fish with mustard mixture, place in a baking dish, cover and refrigerate for 10 minutes to marinate. Remove fish from marinade and place on a baking sheet lightly coated with cooking spray. Sprinkle fish with dill, salt, and pepper. Bake at 350 degrees for 10-12 minutes or until fish flakes eas-ily when tested with fork.

Serves 4

Serving Size: 1 salmon fillet, Calories: 263, Fat: 15 grams, Sodium: 320 mg, Car-bohydrate: 1 grams, Protein: 28 grams.

Desserts and Sweet Snacks

Scottish Oat Cakes

This tasty version of a Scottish favorite makes the house smell amazing as they bake. Eat them with hot tea or top them with a low-sugar fruit spread for dessert.

2 cups quick-cooking oats

½ cup walnuts, finely chopped

½ cup raisins

1 ½ teaspoon cinnamon

1 teaspoon baking powder

Pinch of salt

4 tablespoons margarine, softened

¾ cup lightly-packed light brown sugar

2 large eggs, at room temperature

1 tablespoon distilled white vinegar

2 teaspoons vanilla extract

Preheat oven to 375 degrees. Lightly coat baking sheet with cooking spray. In a medium bowl, combine oats, walnuts, raisins, cinnamon, baking powder, and salt in medium bowl and set aside. In a large bowl, use a hand mixer on medium speed to blend butter and sugar until fluffy, then beat in eggs, then add vinegar and vanilla. Mix in dry ingredients by hand until they are well combined. Drop batter by rounded tablespoon onto the baking sheets, spacing cookies 1 inch apart. Use your fingers to press firmly into flat 2- inch rounds. Bake 7 minutes. Cool for 5 minutes.

Makes 4 dozen cakes/cookies

Serving Size: 1 cookie, Calories: 75, Fat: 3 grams, Sodium: 29 mg, Carbohydrate: 11 grams, Protein: 1 gram

Thai Fried Bananas

Here's a dessert fit for company—and for a splurge, try it with a little low-fat vanilla ice cream or on top of angel food cake. This is actually an easy dish to throw together for a snack, too.

2 tablespoons margarine

4 firm bananas, peeled and cut into 1- inch pieces

¼ cup brown sugar

1 teaspoon black sesame seeds

1 tablespoon lime juice

¼ teaspoon cinnamon

Heat wok over high heat and add margarine. Once melted, add bananas and brown sugar. Stir fry until sugar is dissolved, about 1 minute. Add sesame seeds, lime juice, and cinnamon. Stir fry another 1 minute and serve.

Serves 4

Serving size: 1 cup, Calories: 192, Fat: 3 grams, Sodium: 35 mg, Carbohydrate: 39 grams, Protein: 1 gram

Very Berry Salsa

Love fresh berries in the summer? This salsa has an unexpected flavor that is perfect as a dip with pita chips or tortilla strips and equally delightful over grilled fresh fish.

1 pint blueberries

1 pint strawberries, hulled, sliced

¼ cup sugar or sucralose low-calorie sweetener

3 tablespoons sweet Vidalia onion

1 tablespoon lemon juice

¼ cup toasted slivered almonds

dash of hot sauce (optional)

In a large bowl, combine blueberries, strawberries, sugar, onion, and lemon juice until well coated. Chill for 1 hour. Before serving, add almonds and toss.

Serves 16

Serving Size: ¼ cup, Calories: 42, Carbohydrate: 15 grams, Protein: trace

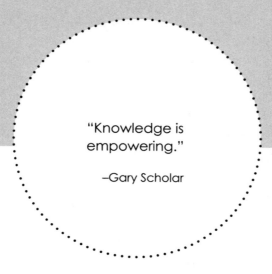

"Knowledge is empowering."

–Gary Scholar

References

American Diabetes Association. (n.d.). *Diabetes basics: Prevention*. Retrieved 17 November 2009 from http://www.diabetes.org/diabetes-basics/prevention/

American Diabetes Association. (n.d.). *Food and fitness*. Retrieved 17 November2009 from http://www.diabetes.org/food-and-fitness/

American Heart Association. (n.d.). *Checklist for lowering your cholesterol*. Retrieved 17 November 2009 from http://www.americanheart.org/presenter.jhtml?identifier=514

American Heart Association. (2008). *Restaurant tips*. Retrieved 21 August 2009 from www.americanheart.org/tips for eating out

American Nurses Association. (2000). *Handle with care fact sheet*. Retrieved 14 December 2009 from http://www.nursingworld.org/MainMenuCategories/OccupationalandEnvironmental/occupationalhealth/handlewithcare/Resources/FactSheet.aspx

Batmanghelidj, F. (1997). *Your body's many cries for water*. Vienna, VA: Global Health Solutions, Inc.

Beattie, M. (1992*). Codependent no more: How to stop controlling others and start caring for yourself.* Center City, MN: Hazelden.

Bogduk, N. (1997). *Clinical anatomy of the lumbar spine and sacrum.* New York: Churchill Livingstone.

Bounchez, C. (2006). *Make the most of your metabolism.* Retrieved 3 August 2009 from http://www.webmd.com/fitness-exercise/guide/make-most-your-metabolism

Chek, P. (1997). *Equal but not the same: Considerations for the female client correspondence course.* Paul Chek Seminars.

Chek, P. (1999). *The golf biomechanics manual: Whole in one golf conditioning.* Vista, CA: C.H.E.K. Institute.

Chek, P. (n.d.). *The importance of ergonomics in rehabilitation.* Retrieved 14 December 2009 from *www.befit2.com/articles/**ErgonomicsCHEK**.pdf*

DonTigny, R. L. (1993). Mechanics and treatment of the sacroiliac joint. *The Journal of Manual and Manipulative Therapy:* 1(1), 3–12.

DonTigny, R. L. (1994). The DonTigny low back pain management program. *The Journal of Manual and Manipulative Therapy,* 2(4), 163–168.

Epstein, L., and Mardon, S. (2007). *The Harvard Medical School guide to a good night's sleep.* Columbus, OH: The McGraw-Hill Companies.

Fox, M. (1998). *Healthy water research.* Retrieved 26 August 2009 from www.healthywater.com.

Glasser, W. (1998). *Choice theory: A new psychology of personal freedom.* New York: HarperCollins Publishers.

Gottaschall, E. (2000). *Breaking the vicious cycle: Intestinal health through diet.* Baltimore, Ontario: Kirkton Press Ltd.

Hitti, M. (2008). *Keeping food diary helps lose weight.* Retrieved 15 July 2009 from www.webMD.com/2008/keeping-food-diary-helps-lose-weight

Hodsdon, W. (2008). *5 ways to prevent depression.* Retrieved 8 September 2009 from http://www.thedietchannel.com/5-Natural-Ways-To-Prevent-Depression.htm

International Journal of Obesity. (2004). Association of weight change, weight control practices, and weight cycling among women in the Nurses Health Study. *Nurses Health Study,* 28, 1134–1142. Retrieved 21 August 2009 from www.nature.com

Jegtvig, S. (2007). *Drinking water to maintain good health.* Retrieved 1 September 2009 from http://nutrition.about .com/od/hydrationwater/a/waterarticle.htm

Kuzemchak, S. (2008). *Outsmarting your cravings.* Retrieved 14 December 2009 from http://www.prevention.com/health/weight-loss/weight-loss-tips/all-about-food-cravings-and-how-to-stop-them/article/478206ef823d6110VgnVCM10000013281eac____/

Laino, C. (2003). *Is PMS sabotaging your diet?* Retrieved 14 December 2009 from http://www.webmd.com/diet/features/is-pms-sabotaging-your-diet

Mayo Clinic. (2008). *High blood pressure (hypertension): Lifestyle and home remedies.* Retrieved 17 November 2009 from http://www.mayoclinic.com/health/high-blood-pressure/DS00100/DSECTION=lifestyle-and-home-remedies

McLaughlin, M. (2007). *Self-care for back pain: Caring for a bad back.* Retrieved 14 December 2009 from http://northridgehospital.staywellsolutionsonline.com/Wellness/Backand-Neck/Dealing/Selfcare/1,4146

Mercola, J. (n.d.). *The beginner nutrition plan.* Retrieved 27 August 2009 from www.mercola.com/nutritionplan/beginner.htm.

National Eating Disorders Association. (2009a). *Terms and definitions.* Retrieved 19 September 2009 from http://www.nationaleatingdisorders.org/information-resources/general-information.php#terms-definitions

National Eating Disorders Association. (2009b). *Factors that may contribute to eating disorders.* Retrieved 14 December 2009 from http://www.nationaleatingdisorders.org/information-resources/general-information.php#causes-eating-disorders

Nightingale, F. (1860). *Notes on nursing.* New York: D. Appleton & Company.

Northrup, C. (2006). *The wisdom of menopause: Creating physical and emotional health during the change.* New York: The Bantam Dell Publishing Group.

Nurses' Health Study Annual Newsletter. (2002). *Physical activity.* Retrieved 4 August 2009 from www.channing.harvard.edu/nhs/newsletters/pds/n2002.pdf

Nurses' Health Study Annual Newsletter. (2005). *Sugar sweetened beverages weight gain and diabetes risk.* Retrieved 4 August 2009 from www.channing.harvard.edu/nhs/newsletters/pds/n2005.pdf

Nurses' Health Study Annual Newsletter. (2007). *Trans fats banned for good reason.* Retrieved 4 August 2009 from www.channing.harvard.edu/nhs/newsletters/pdf/n2007.pdf

Pollan, M. (2009). *Healthcare crisis.* Georgia Organics Conference, March 21, 2009. Retrieved 2 December 2009 from http://www.mnn.com/lifestyle/health/videos/michael-pollan-healthcare-crisis

Querna, B. (2005). Stopping PMS: Calcium and vitamin D could help prevent PMS. *U.S. News & World Report.* Retrieved 3 December 2009 from http://health.usnews.com/usnews/health/briefs/nutrition/hb050614a.htm

Rajaram, S., Haddad, E., Mejia, A., and Sabate, J. (2009). Walnuts and fatty fish influence different serum lipid fractions. *American Journal of Clinical Nutrition* (electronic version), 89(5), 1657s–1663s.

Richardson, C. (2009). *The art of extreme self-care: Transform your life one month at a time.* Carlsbad, CA: Hay House, Inc.

Seaman, D. (1998). *Clinical nutrition: For pain, inflammation, and tissue healing.* Greenville, SC: NutrAnalysis, Inc.

Vleeming, A., Mooney, V., & Stoeckart, R. (2007). Functional control of the spine. In Movement, stability, and lumbopelvic pain: *Integration of research and therapy.* New York: Churchill Livingstone, 489–512.

WebMD. (2007). *Cholesterol management guide: Take steps to reduce cholesterol.* Retrieved 17 November 2009 from http://www.webmd.com/cholesterol-management/guide/steps-to-reduce-cholesterol

WebMD. (2008). *Diet for depression.* Retrieved 7 December 2009 from http://www.webmd.com/depression/guide/diet-recovery

WebMD. (2008). *Exercise and depression.* Retrieved 7 December 2009 from http://www.webmd.com/depression/guide/exercise-depression

WebMD. (n.d.). *Hypertension/high blood pressure guide: Treatment & care.* Retrieved 17 November 2009 from http://www.webmd.com/hypertension-high-blood-pressure/guide/

WebMD. (n.d.). *Premenstrual syndrome (PMS): treatment overview.* Retrieved 3 December 2009 from http://women.webmd.com/pms/premenstrual-syndrome-pms-treatment-overview

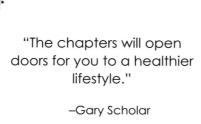

"The chapters will open doors for you to a healthier lifestyle."

–Gary Scholar

Index

A

abdominal canister, 88
accomplishments, 20
accountability, fitness plan, 53
activities one enjoys, 50
acupuncture, 97
adipocytes, 38
age, metabolism and, 32
alcohol, blood pressure and, 40–41
alertness, exercise and, 53
American Diabetes Association, 37
    exercise advice, 55–56
American Heart Association, 37

anorexia nervosa, 159, 160
anti-inflammatory foods, 84
assertiveness, 20–21
    accountability weight loss progress, 149
    believing in oneself, 21
    boundary setting, 25–27
    codependency and, 21
    examples, 27–28
    implementing, 24
    job performance and, 22–23
    looping and, 24
    scheduling exercise, 53
    weight management, 150

B

back
  neutral spine, 92–93
  strengthening, 90–91
back pain
  causes, 80
  clinical instability, 86
  disc pain, 86
  DonTigny seated knee reach
    sacroiliac joint mobilization, 94
  ergonomics and, 90
  feet and, 83
  four-point transversus abdominus
    activation trainer, 92–94
  horse stance, 94
  hydration and, 84
  lifestyle and, 84
  managing, 87–89
  massage therapy, 82–83
  muscles strengthened, 88–89
  origins, 88
  sacroiliac joint pain, 87
  sleep and, 90
  spinal stenosis, 85
  spondylolisthesis, 85–86
  stress and, 99
  Swiss ball
    forward ball roll, 96–97
    hip extension, 95
    seated posture trainer, 95–96
  TCM (Traditional Chinese Medi-
    cine), 97–100
  weight and, 81
bakery shopping, 198
Barret, Dr. Max, 83
Beattie, Melody (*Codependent No More*),
  4
BED (binge eating disorder), 159, 160
beef, grass-fed, 200
believing in oneself, 21
Bielak, Maia, 82

binge eating, 104
  binge eating disorder, 159, 160
biometric screening, 180
blood pressure, 37
  alcohol, 40–41
  body fat, 38
  dehydration, 42
  exercise, 40, 54
  fats, 40
  healthy, 38–42
  insomnia, 41
  medication, 41
  nuts, 39–40
  optimum blood pressure, 38
  salt intake, 38
  smoking, 41
  sodium, 39
  stress management, 41
  water intake, 42
blood sugar
  comfort eating, 106–109
  desserts, 107
  eating every 3-4 hours, 107
  exercise, 54
  foods, 44–45
  glycemic index, 115
BMI (body mass index), 3, 38
BMR (basal metabolic rate), 32
body, listening to, 153–155
body composition, metabolism and, 32
body fat, 38
boredom eating, 104
boundary setting, 25–27
boxing techniques, 74–75
breakfast, weight management and, 150
bulimia nervosa, 159, 160
burnout, overcare, 6–7

C

caffeine, 2, 125
  night shift nurses, 136
  reducing, 115–116
calories burned, 32
canned goods, 201
carbs
  complex, 121
  refined, 121
cardio fitness, 62
care plans
  fitness charting, 191
  nutrition charting, 186–189
career impact on weight management,
  151
Caring for the Caregiver Therapeutic
  Massage Program, 82
cereals, 201–202
challenges
  food, 8–9
  overwhelmed feelings, 19
  shift work, 7–8
  stress, 9–10
  Type E personality, 5–7
channels (TCM), 166
charting goals, 17–18
Childers, Raina RD, 128, 158
children respecting parents' need for
  self care, 14
Children's Memorial Hospital (Chicago), 82
Chinese herbs, 99
ChiWalking, 59
choice, Lifestyle Shift and, 3
Choice Theory (Glasser), 4
cholesterol, 37
  exercise, 42, 54
  fats, 42, 43
  fiber, 43
  HDL, 42
  LDL, 42
  numbers, 42

Omega 3 fats, 42
  smoking, 44
  stress management, 44
  sugar, 42
  triglycerides, 42
chronic back pain, 85
circadian rhythms, shift work and, 7
clinical instability, 86
Code Blue foods, 123–125, 202–203
Code Emerald foods, 123–125, 197
  bakery, 198
  deli, 200
  meat, 199–200
  produce, 198
Code Gray Program, 157
codependency, assertiveness and, 21
Codependent No More (Beattie), 4
coffee. *See* caffeine
comfort eating
  effects of, 107
  location of food, 105–106
  reasons, 104–105
  SCRUBS (Sugar Cravings Ruin
    Blood Sugar), 106–109
comfort food
  addictive nature of, 108
  binge eating, 104
  cortisol and, 33
  discharging, 109–111, 114–115
  effects of, 107
  exchange, 116
  healthy, 196
  serotonin, 108
  in work environment, 104, 105–106
commitment to fitness, 48
compassion fatigue, 6
complex carbs, 121
concierge service, 182
core, strengthening, 90–91
cortisol
  exercise and, 48
  food cravings and, 33
  stress and, 32–33

CSA (community supported agriculture), 196
cupping, 98
Curves, 61

D

daily choices, changing, 14
dairy, 202
death of patient, coping with, 156–158
deceleration after work, 7
dehydration, blood pressure and, 42
deli shopping, 200
depression, foods and, 127–128
deprivation, overgiving and, 7
deserving to feel healthier, 6
desserts, 107
diabetes, 37
    exercise and, 55–56
    glycemic index and, 115
dietary fiber, 121
dieting, yo-yo dieting, 33
digestion, TCM, 168
dining out, 132
DonTigny seated knee reach sacroiliac joint mobilization, 94
DVD workouts, 65

E

eating
    experience of, 168–169
    schedule for night shift nurses, 142
    toothpaste technique, 154
eating disorders
    causes, 161
    coping with, 158–159
    symptoms, 160
e

motions
    death of a patient, 156–158
    weight management and, 150
empowered fitness, 61–62
empowerment, 10
encouragement, 5
endorphins, exercise and, 48
energy expenditure (metabolism), 32
energy level, exercise and, 49
Energy Plate, 122–123
Epstein, Lawrence (*The Harvard Medical School Guide to a Good Night's Sleep*), 143
ergonomics, 90
excuses, 4
exercise. *See also* fitness
    alertness and, 53
    back pain and, 80
    benefits, 53–54
    blood pressure, 40, 54
    blood sugar, 54
    boxing techniques, 74–75
    cardio fitness, 62
    care plans, 56–65
    cholesterol, 42, 54
    cortisol and, 48
    Curves, 61
    diabetes and, 55–56
    dropouts, 50
    DVD workouts, 65
    endorphins, 48
    energy level and, 48–49
    enjoyable, 49–50
    flexibility, 59–60, 62
    fun activities, 65
    interval training, 59
    metabolism and, 48
    muscle tension and, 54
    rewards, 148
    scheduling, 50, 51–52
        12-hour shift, 65–66
        night shift, 66
        traveling nurses, 66–67

strength training, 60–61, 63–65, 76–78
stress and, 48, 53
Tai Chi, 67–71
time for, 48
walking, 58–59
weight management and, 53, 150
yoga/Pilates, 71–74
exercise ball, 60–61
back alignment at desk, 82
expectations, guilt and, 25
expressing needs, 26

F

F-I-N-E (Frequently Ignoring Needs and Emotions), 25
family
dealing with, 176–177
ripple effect through, 177
fast foods/slow foods, 34–35
fatigue, compassion fatigue, 6
fats
blood pressure, 40
cholesterol, 42, 43
monounsaturated fats, 121
polyunsaturated fats, 121
saturated, 119
trans fats, 121, 122
fatty fish, 121
feet, back pain and, 83
fiber, 121
cholesterol, 43
fish, mercury in, 198
fitness. *See also* exercise
accountability, 53
boxing techniques, 74–75
cardio, 62
charting in care plan, 191
commitment to, 48
Curves, 61
DVD workouts, 65

empowered, 61–62
enjoyable exercise, 49–50
fun activities, 65
interval training, 59
reasons for, 48
scheduling
12-hour shift, 65–66
night shift, 66
traveling nurses, 66–67
self-esteem and, 48
strength training, 60–61, 63–65, 76–78
Tai Chi, 67–71
yoga/Pilates, 71–74
flexibility exercises, 59–60, 62
food, 8–9. *See also* comfort food; nutrition
anti-inflammatory foods, 84
bakery, 198
canned goods, 201
cereals, 201–202
Code Blue, 123–125, 202–203
Code Emerald, 123–125, 197
cravings, cortisol and, 33
dairy, 202
deli, 200
depression and, 127–128
diary, 120, 190
digestion (TCM), 168
frozen food, 202
hospital cafeteria, 125–127
inflammatory foods, 84
label reading, 194–195
local, 169–170, 196
meat, 199–200
menus, 130–131
night shift, 140–141
oils, 200
organic, 169
portion control, 122–123
prepackaged, 201
produce, 198
rice/pasta, 201

salad dressings, 201
seafood, 198–199
in season, 167
sleep and, 142–143
soft drinks, 109
TCM and, 167–170
weighing, 129, 139
four-point transversus abdominus activation trainer, 92–94
friends
 dealing with, 176–177
 ripple effect through, 177
frozen food, 202

G

G-U-I-L-T (Guaranteeing You Infinite Lifetime Therapy), 25
GERD (gastroesophageal reflux disease), 136
Glasser, Dr. William *(Choice Theory)*, 4
glycemic index, 115
goals, charting, 17–18
Golden Nightingale Wings, 179–180
grass-fed beef, 200
grieving, 157
grocery shopping, 116
guilt, 7
 origins and, 25

H–I

HDL (high-density lipoprotein) cholesterol, 42
Health Point Fitness, 128
healthy comfort foods, 196
heart rate
 raising, 49
 target, 54–55

heroes, 182
holistic health, 164. *See also* TCM (Traditional Chinese Medicine)
 nurse lifestyle, 164–165
honesty with self, 6
hormones, cholesterol, 42
horse stance, 94
Hospice Foundation of America, 158
hospital cafeteria, 125–127
Hungry Girl Web site, 133
hydration, back pain and, 84
hypnosis, 152
hypothyroidism, 34

I Bet I Can Plan, 181–182
I WIN bracelet, 111–112
 knitting pattern, 112–113
inflammatory foods, 84
insomnia, blood pressure and, 41
interval training, 59

J–K–L

job performance, assertiveness and, 22–23
Johnson, Michelle, 82

Kimball, Molly R.D., 34
kitchen scales, 129, 139
knitting pattern for I WIN bracelet, 112–113
Kuzemchak, Sally, R.D., 32–33

label reading, 194–195
lamenectomy, 81
LDL (low-density lipoprotein) cholesterol, 3, 42
lifestyle
 back pain and, 84
 current *versus* optimal, 15–18
 as food plate, 14–18
 holistic approach, 164–165

Lifestyle Shift, 1
    choice and, 3
    reasons for starting, 14
    stress levels, 2
Lillien, Lisa, 133
listening to your body, 153–155
living well as best medicine, 2
local food, 169–170, 196
location of food, comfort eating and, 105–106
long-term weight management, 150–151
long working hours, 7
looping, 23–24
    assertiveness and, 24–25
    author's, 25
    perfectionism and, 153

M

Mardon, Steven (*The Harvard Medical School Guide to a Good Night's Sleep*), 143
massage therapy, 82–83
Mayo Clinic, 37
meals
    planning, 129
        night shift nurses, 136–137, 138
        shopping for food and, 196
    skipping, 33
meat, shopping for, 199–200
meditation, 170
    stress reduction and, 99
melatonin, 90
menus, 130–131
    night shift, 140–141
mercury in fish, 198
meridians (TCM), 166
metabolism
    age and, 32
    BMR (basal metabolic rate), 32
    body composition and, 32

cholesterol, 42
    definition, 32
    energy expenditure, 32
    exercise and, 48
    extra weight and, 34
    hypothyroidism, 34
    natural ways to boost and balance, 35–36
    night shift nurses, 136
    PAEE (physical activity energy expenditure), 32
    as patient, 31
    sleep and, 143
    starving oneself and, 149
    TEF (thermic effect of food), 32
    yo-yo dieting and, 33
microdisketomy, 81
mobile munchies, 137–138
monounsaturated fats, 121
mothers, 6
moxibustion (TCM), 99
multitasking, stress and, 4, 26
muscle tension, exercise and, 54

N

NEDA (National Eating Disorders Association), 159
needs, expressing, 26
neutral spine, 92–93
Night Shift Committee, 144–145
night shift menus, 140–141
night shift nurses, 7, 135
    caffeine, 136
    eating habits, 9
    eating schedule, 142
    GERD, 136
    meal planning, 136–137
    metabolism, 136
    mobile munchies, 137–138
    sleep, 136, 142–143
    sleep deprivation, 143

Nightingale, Florence, "nature acting upon patient," 11
Nightingale Living Well Pledge, 152, 153
Nightingale Pledge, 152
Nightingale Wellness Bucks, 181–182
North Shore Physical Wellness, 83
Northrup, Christiane (*The Wisdom of Menopause*)
  self-sacrifice, 6
  toxic stress/toxic weight gain, 33
nurse
  glycemic, 106
  as patient, 171–172
  as theater director, 4
nutrition. *See also* food
  anti-inflammatory foods, 84
  back pain and, 84
  carbs
    complex, 121
    refined, 121
  charting in care plan, 186–189
  Chinese, 164
  eat every 3-4 hours, 107
  fiber, 121
  food diary, 120
  hospital cafeteria, 125–127
  inflammatory foods, 84
  monounsaturated fats, 121
  planning meals, 129
  polyunsaturated fats, 121
  portion control, 122–123
  restaurants, 132
  saturated fats, 119
  trans fat, 121, 122
nuts, 39–40

O

OA (Overeaters Anonymous), 159
oils, 200
Okinawa Program, 43

Omega 3 fats, 44, 121
  cholesterol, 42
Omega 6 fats, 121
organic food, 169
orthopedic injuries, 85
overcare, 6–7
overgiving, 7
overwhelmed feelings, overcoming, 20

P-Q

PAEE (physical activity energy expenditure), 32
pain
  acute, 85
  chronic, 85
  trigger points, 91
Palicka, Donna, 111–112
paradigm shift, 10
patient's death, coping with, 156–158
pedometer, 58
  steps per day, 59
perfectionism, 153–154
Pilates, 71–74
planning, 11
  meals, 129
    night shift nurses, 138
    shopping for food and, 196
  night shift nurses, 136–137
plateau in workout, interval training, 59
PMS, 108
polyunsaturated fats, 121
portion control, 122–123
positive encouragement, 5
prepackaged food, 201
prioritizing self care, 6
processed foods, fast foods, 35
produce, shopping for, 198

Qi (TCM), 98, 166
questions to ask self, 6

R

recipes
  appetizers and snacks
    Baked Tortilla Strips, 206–207
    Five-Pepper Hummus, 205–206
    Southwest Snack Mix, 206
  desserts and sweet snacks
    Scottish Oat Cakes, 234
    Thai Fried Bananas, 235
    Very Berry Salsa, 235
  meat main dishes
    Asian Beef Steaks and Noodles, 228
    Baked Chicken Tortillas, 229
    Baked Salmon with Lemon-Dill Mustard Sauce, 233
    Homestyle Meatloaf, 230
    Italian Chicken with Garlic and Chickpeas, 231
    Pork Chops with Apple-Pear Chutney, 232
  salads
    Blackened Portobello Mushroom Salad, 210
    Citrus Chicken and Soba Noodle Salad, 211
    Jicama and Fruit Salad, 213–214
    Mediterranean Chicken Salad, 212
    Roasted Pepper, Wax Bean, and Tomato Salad, 217
    Shrimp Salad with Pineapple and Pecans, 213
    Spicy Asian Slaw, 214
    Springtime Fruit Salad with Citrus-Mint Dressing, 215
    Summertime Black-Eyed Pea Salad, 215–216
    Vegetarian Tuscan Salad, 216
  soups
    Chicken Tortilla Soup, 207
    Chunky Sausage, Corn and Habanero Chili, 208
    Squash-Quinoa Soup, 209
  vegetables and side dishes
    Asparagus with Lemon and Mustard, 219–220
    Basil Roasted Vegetables with Couscous, 220
    Cajun-Style Collard Greens, 218
    Pine Nut Topped Green Beans, 219
  vegetarian main dishes
    Artichoke Omelet, 224
    Asparagus Tomato Stir Fry, 221
    Black Bean and Spinach Pizza, 222
    Egg Fried Rice, 223
    Greek Stuffed Eggplant, 225
    Tofu, Asparagus, and Red Pepper Stir-Fry with Quinoa, 226
    Vegetable Pie Mexicana, 227
red scarf as signal to family, 7
Redmond, Karen MS, 81
refined carbs, 121
relaxation techniques, 41
  back pain and, 99
resistance bands, 60–61
responsibility for self, 148
restaurant dining, 132
restrictive diets, 149
rewards, 148
rice/pasta, 201
Richardson, Cheryl (*The Art of Extreme Self-Care*), 7
Roessler, Ryan, 152
Roswell Park Cancer Institute (Buffalo), 157

S

sabotage by friends/family, 176
sacrifice, Type E personality, 5

sacroiliac joint pain, 87
salt, table salt *versus* sea salt, 39
satisfaction, Type E personality, 5
saturated fats, 119
scales, 129, 139
scheduling exercise, 50, 51–52
    12-hour shift, 65–66
    night shift, 66
    traveling nurses, 66–67
SCRUBS (Sugar Cravings Ruin Blood Sugar), 106–109
sea salt, 39
seafood, shopping for, 198–199
Second Shift Syndrome, 7–8
self-awareness, 6
self care
    children respecting need for, 14
    as priority, 6
    self-awareness, 6
    silent epidemic of denial, 4
    TCM (Traditional Chinese Medicine), 170
self-esteem, fitness and, 48
serotonin, comfort foods, 108
Shaping up with Weights for Dummies, 60
shift gears after work, 7
shift work, 7–8
    eating habits, 9
shoes, 57
shopping for food, 116
    bakery, 198
    canned goods, 201
    cereals, 201–202
    dairy, 202
    expense, 203
    frozen food, 202
    full stomach, 198
    label reading, 194–195
    lists, 196
    meat, 199–200
    oils, 200
    power shopping, 196–203
    prepackaged foods, 201
    produce, 198
    rice/pasta, 201
    salad dressings, 201
    seafood, 198–199
significance, Type E personality, 5
silent epidemic of denying self care, 4
Sister-Arts Studio (Chicago), 111–112
skipped meals, 33
sleep
    back pain and, 90
    food and, 142–143
    looping and, 23
    metabolism and, 143
    night shift nurses, 136, 142–143
    sleep deprivation, 143
smoking
    blood pressure and, 41
    cholesterol, 44
snacks, 137–138
sodium, 39
soft drinks, 109, 125
Southeast Missouri Hospital, 128
spinal stenosis, 85
spondylolisthesis, 85–86
start date target, 148
starving oneself, 149
steps per day, 59
strength training, 60–61, 63–65, 76–78
    exercise ball, 60–61
    resistance bands, 60–61
stress
    back pain and, 99
    challenge to lifestyle, 2
    cortisol, 32–33
    eating disorders, 158–161
    exercise and, 48, 53
    looping and, 23
    managing
        blood pressure and, 41
        cholesterol, 44

multitasking, 4
toxic stress/toxic weight gain, 33
stressors, 9–10
 death of patient, 156–158
 multitasking, 26
stretching, back pain, 80
subconscious mind and weight management, 152
success at weight loss, programming
 for, 149
sugar
 cholesterol, 42
 names for on labels, 194
support team, sabotage, 176
Suzuki, Makoto MD, 43
Swiss balls, 61
 back alignment at desk, 82
 forward ball roll, 96–97
 hip extension, 95
 seated posture trainer, 95–96

T

Tai Chi, 67–71
target heart rate, 54–55
target start date, 148
TCM (Traditional Chinese Medicine),
 97–99
 back pain, 97–100
 balance, 164
 body, mind, spirit, 165
 branch, 164
 channel, 166
 Chinese herbs, 99
 digestion, 168
 eating experience, 168–169
 food
  flavors, 167
  local, 169–170
  organic, 169

 properties, 167
 in season, 167
Gua sha, 99
holistic approach to lifestyle,
 164–165
holistic perspective, 164
meridian, 166
moxibustion, 99
nutrition, 164
Qi, 166
root, 164
self care, 170
Tui na, 99
whole person, 163
yin/yang, 166
TEF (thermic effect of food), 32
The Art of Extreme Self-Care (Richardson), 7
*The Harvard Medical School Guide to
 a Good Night's Sleep* (Epstein and
 Mardon), 143
The Wisdom of Menopause (Northrup),
 6
toothpaste technique, 154
toxic stress/toxic weight gain, 33
Traditional Chinese Medicine (TCM),
 97–99
trans fat, 121, 122
treadmill, 58
trigger points for pain management,
 91
triglycerides, 42
Tui na (TCM), 99
TVA (transversus abdominis), 88
Type E personality
 development stages, 5–6
 payoff, 5
 sacrifice, 5

W

walking
  ChiWalking, 59
  form, 58
  pedometer, 58
    steps per day, 59
  on shift, 49
  treadmill, 58
walnuts, 121
water intake
  blood pressure and, 42
  flavoring, 41
  types, 129, 139
WebMD, 37
weighing food, 129, 139
weight
  back pain and, 81
  cycling, 34
  loss
    assertiveness accountability
      weight loss progress, 149
    Chinese nutrition, 169
    rate, 148
    starving oneself, 149
    success, programming for, 149
  management, 33–34
    breakfast, 150
    career impact on, 151
    emotions, 150
    exercise and, 53
    long-term, 150–151
    subconscious mind and, 152
wellness challenge, 178–179
  awards presentation, 181
Wellsprings Hypnosis (Chicago), 152
Willcox, Bradley MD, 43
Willcox, Craig PhD, 43
work environment
  comfort food in, 104, 105–106
  health eating and, 106
working hours, long, 7
worry, looping, 23

X–Y–Z

yin/yang energy (TCM), 98–99, 166
yo-yo dieting, 33
yoga, 71–74

Books by, for, and about nurses from the Honor Society of Nursing, Sigma Theta Tau International

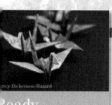

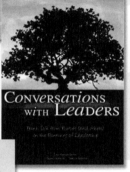

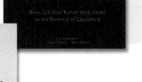

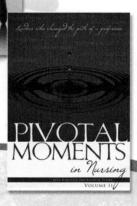

True to STTI's vision, the honor society's nursing publications support the growth of a global community of nurses who lead using scholarship, knowledge, and technology to improve the health of the world's people.

PUBLISHED BY:

Sigma Theta Tau International
Honor Society of Nursing®

DISTRIBUTED BY:

nursing **KNOWLEDGE**
international®

Order your copies today at
www.nursingknowledge.org/STTI/books

Be inspired daily with daybooks from the Honor Society of Nursing, Sigma Theta Tau International

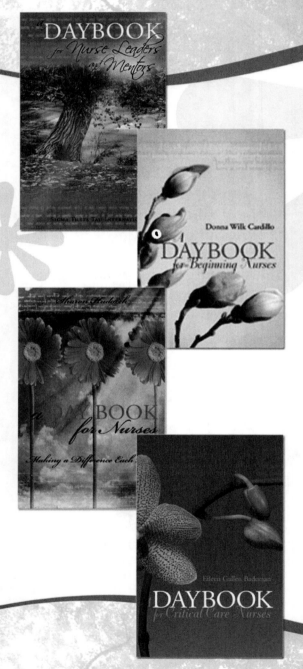

These daily motivational books provide inspiration nurses as they strive to make a difference in the lives of the patients, families, and communities they serve.

PUBLISHED BY:

Sigma Theta Tau International
Honor Society of Nursing

DISTRIBUTED BY:

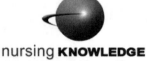

nursing **KNOWLEDGE**
international

Order your copies today at
www.nursingknowledge.org/STTI/books